Christmas 2000

To Sharon

Best wishes to you for a
healthy pregnancy,

with love

Fiona & Jon
XX

P.S. Happy Christmas!

PREGNANCY

A WEEK-BY-WEEK GUIDE

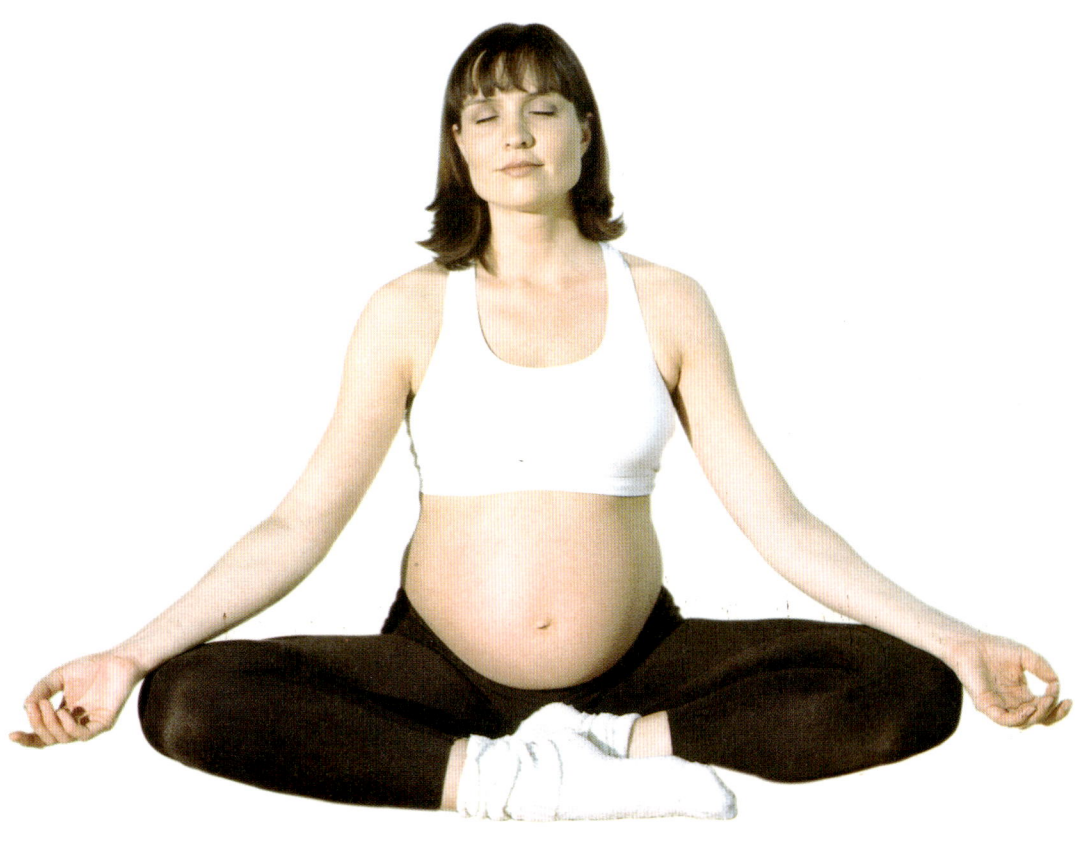

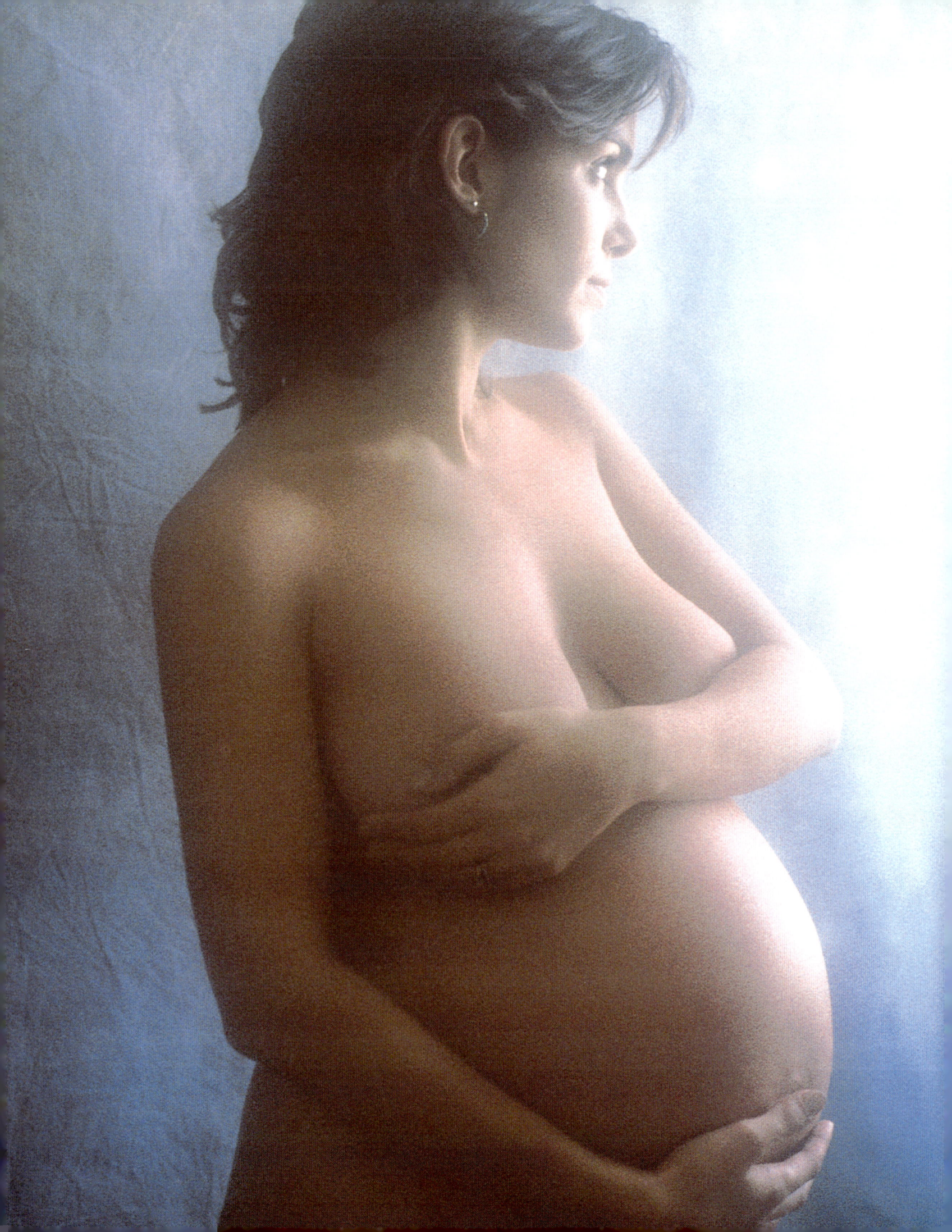

PREGNANCY

A WEEK-BY-WEEK GUIDE

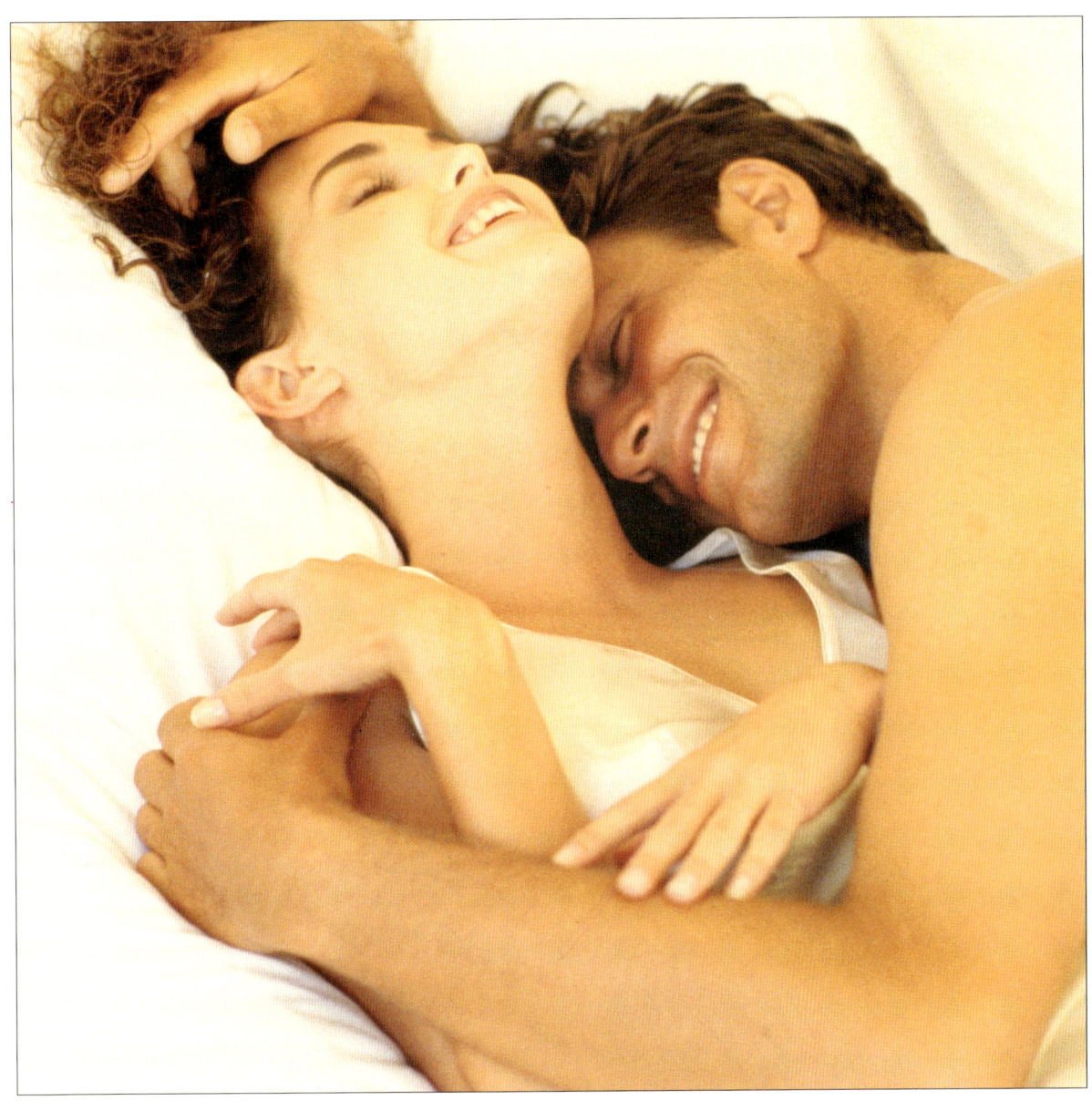

DAN BROMAGE

EDITED BY RICHARD EMERSON

ABBEYDALE PRESS

Published by Abbeydale Press
An imprint of
Bookmart Limited
Registered Number 2372865
Trading as Bookmart Limited
Desford Road
Enderby
Leicester
LE9 5AD

ISBN 1-86147-044-4

Produced for Bookmart by Stonecastle Graphics Limited

Printed in Spain

Photograph/illustration credits:
(Abbreviations t = top, b = below, l = left, r = right, c = centre)

© Telegraph Colour Library: Pages 1, 2, 3, 6br, 7t, 8t, 9b, 10, 11, 12, 13, 14b, 16, 17, 18, 21b, 22, 23r, 24l, 26t, 30tl, 33b, 34t, 40, 41, 43, 44b, 46t, 47, 49t, 49c, 50t, 51br, 53t, 54, 55, 56t, 57r, 62b, 65t, 69t, 69r, 70r, 70b, 72l, 72b, 74l, 77, 78t, 80l, 81, 82t, 86, 88, 91t.

© Eddie Lawrence: Pages 6t, 9r, 14t, 19, 24r, 25t, 30bl, 32, 33t, 34b, 35b, 42b, 52, 56l, 57t, 61b, 62t, 63, 64, 65br, 65bl, 70tl, 71, 74t, 74c, 75t, 75l, 75c, 76t, 80t, 82b, 83, 84t, 85, 87, 89t, 89bl, 90, 91b, 94t.

© Touchstone: Pages 23, 25b, 49b, 73, 75b.

Medical illustrations © Sean Milne: Pages 15, 17r, 25, 29, 33, 35, 41, 43, 47, 51, 53, 55t, 59, 61, 67, 69, 75, 77, 81, 83, 85b, 87.

Medical Editor: Dr Carol Cooper
Consultant Medical Editor: Dr J Sanger

CONTENTS

*I*NTRODUCTION

*W*ELCOME TO 'Pregnancy – A Week-By-Week Guide'. You are about to embark on an incredible journey... Congratulations on buying a book that will act as your guide and source of information during this important time in your life.

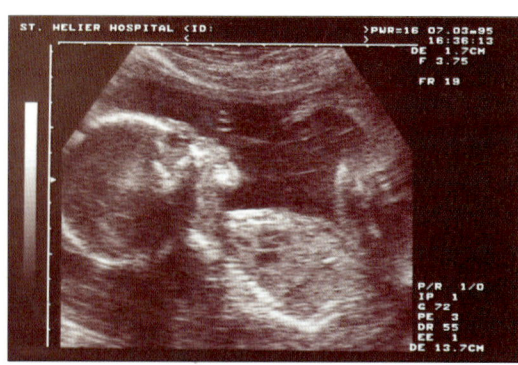

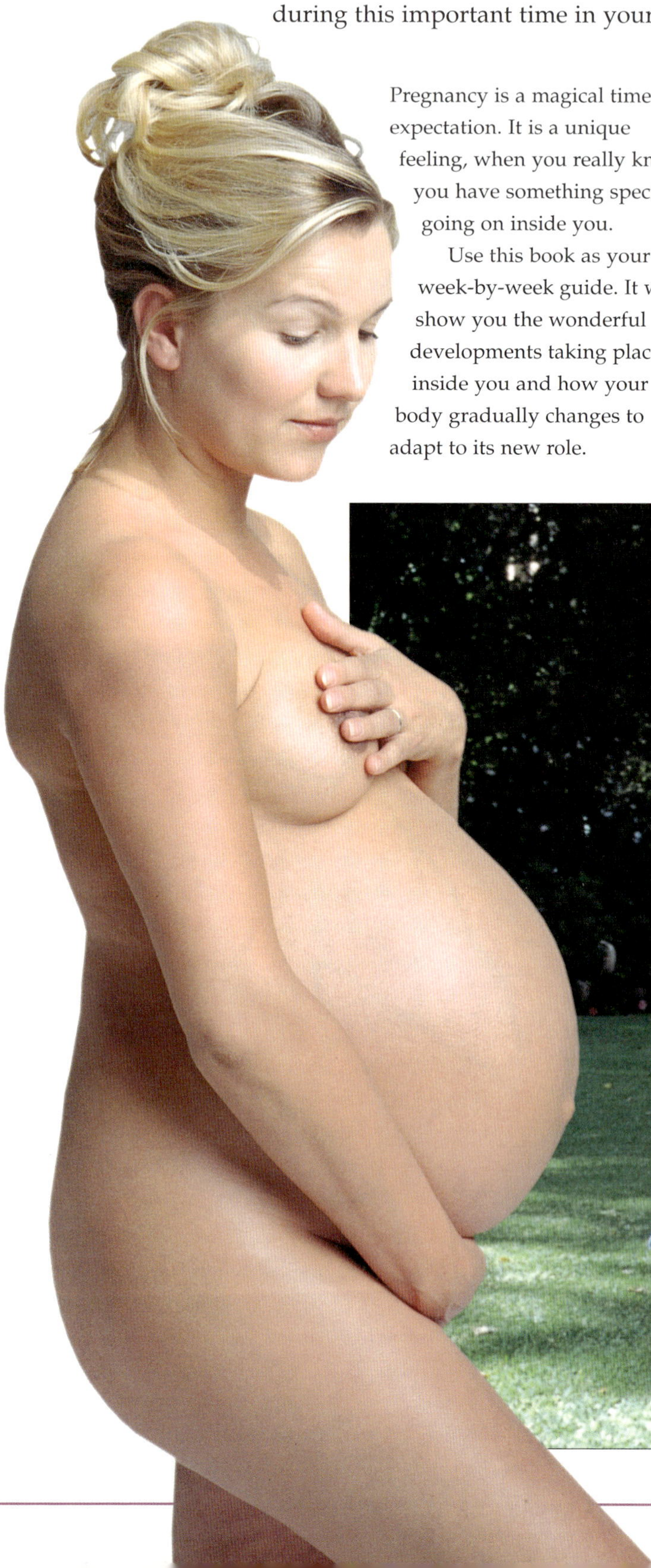

Pregnancy is a magical time of expectation. It is a unique feeling, when you really know you have something special going on inside you.

Use this book as your week-by-week guide. It will show you the wonderful developments taking place inside you and how your body gradually changes to adapt to its new role.

This is also a crucial time for you and your baby. Keeping yourself healthy is so important to the wellbeing of your child – many adult health problems can be traced to the mother's health during pregnancy. For instance, smoking during pregnancy is known to be linked to premature or low birthweight babies, and may also contribute to a whole host of other problems including childhood and adult asthma.

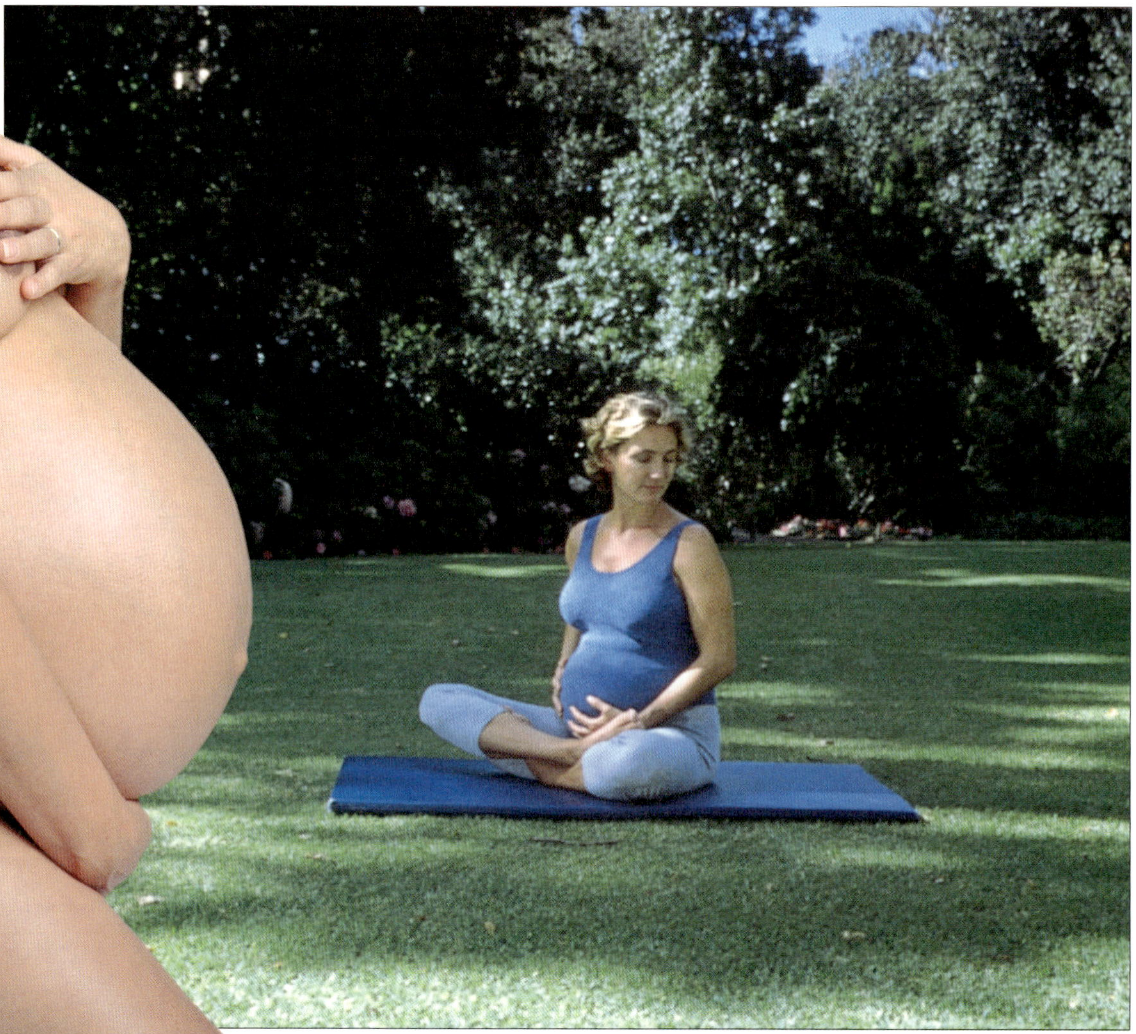

Staying happy and well during your nine months of pregnancy also involves a good diet, exercise and relaxation. The expectant mother should know about the importance of nutrients like folic acid and iron; why she will feel more fatigued at the beginning and end of her pregnancy; and how exercise

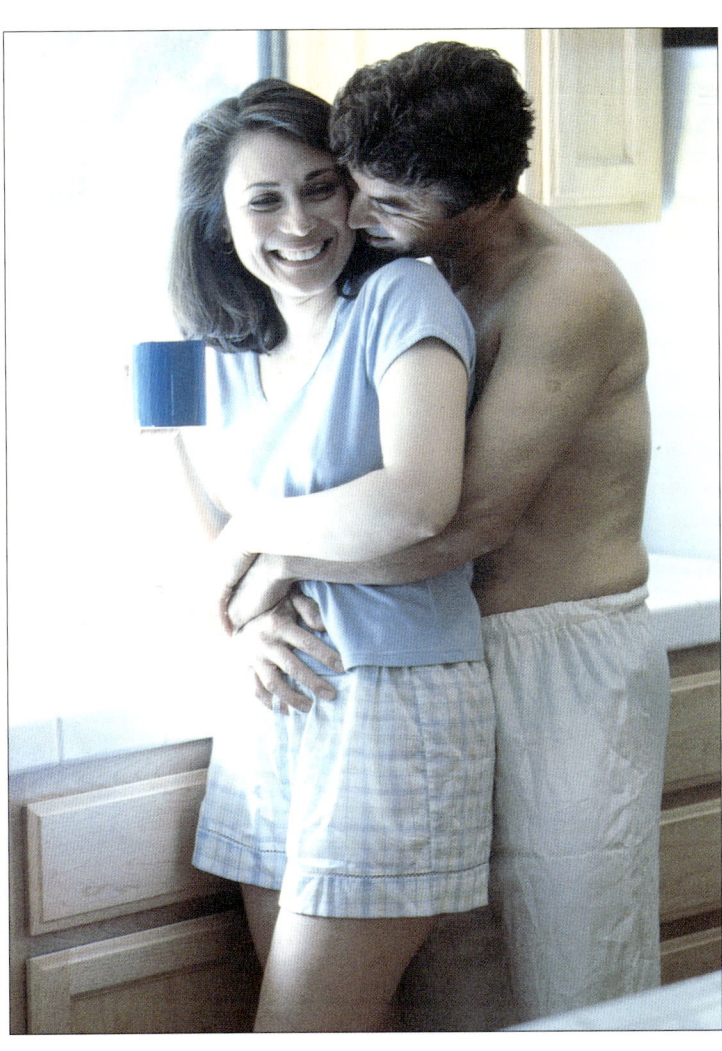

will help her enjoy pregnancy and recover more quickly after the birth. She needs to know the strong emotional effects pregnancy can have on her and her partner, and that her feelings are part and parcel of the whole process. After all, what could possibly be more intense and exhilarating than having a child, whether you're the mother or the father?

There are always the people in white coats to think about, too. In our age of managed healthcare, we have achieved remarkable feats in reducing infant mortality and improving the wellbeing and choices of parents during pregnancy, birth and infant care. This means you'll be seeing rather a lot of your midwife and doctor over the next few months. This book

will explain when you'll be visiting, what they will ask of you and how this will affect your pregnancy. We also look at the process of birth, your birth and pain relief choices, and how you can make the experience a rewarding and fulfilling one.

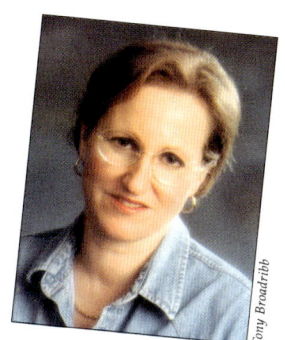

Carol Cooper

Dr Carol Cooper

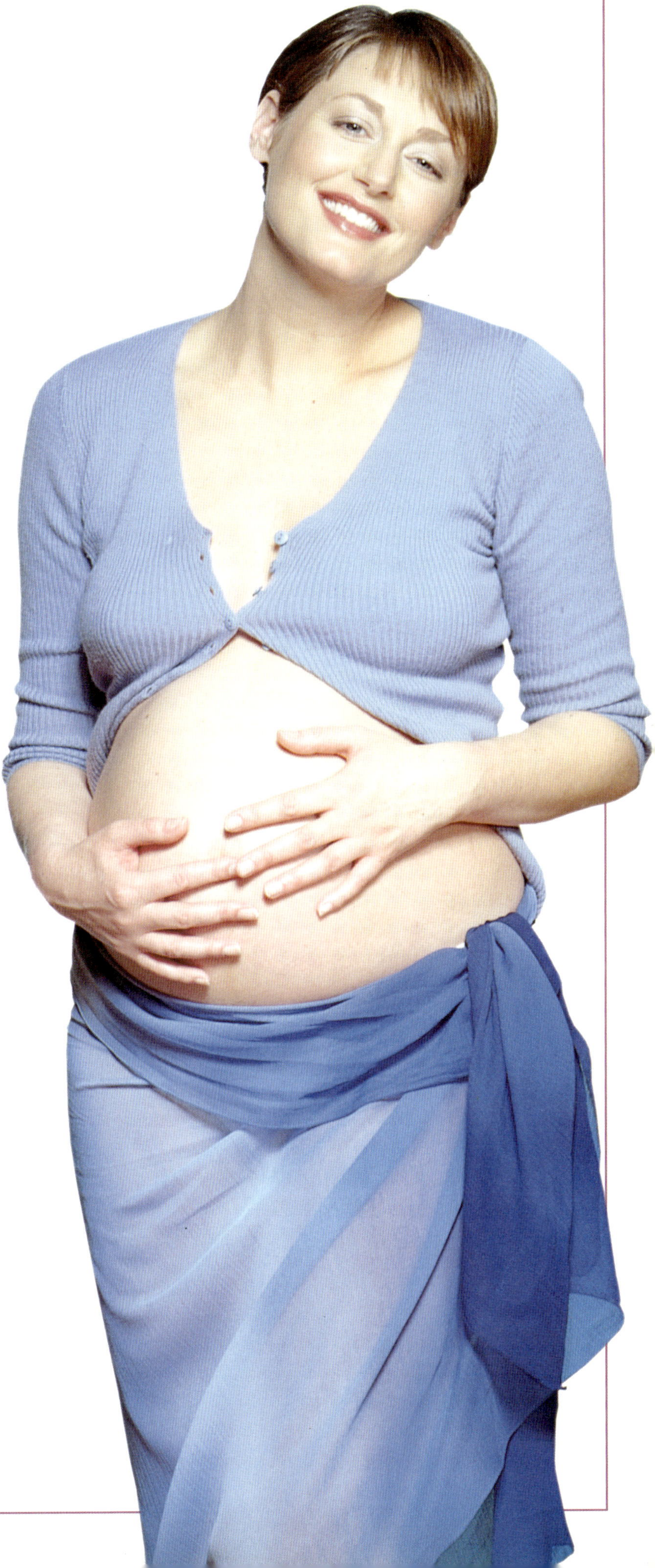

FIT AND FERTILE

ONCE YOU know the processes involved in reproduction, and the factors that can affect your fertility and that of your partner, you can take steps to improve your chances of conceiving. On the following pages, there will be more information and advice to help you have a problem-free pregnancy and labour – and a healthy baby.

Of the 400 million sperm your partner ejaculates during sex, only one will actually enter and fertilise the egg.

During your reproductive life, you will release 400–500 eggs (or ova) from your ovaries, a process known as ovulation. Most months, one egg will travel along one of your uterine tubes (also known as fallopian tubes). If the egg encounters a sperm that is able to penetrate its outer layer, fertilisation will then occur.

Natural selection

During intercourse, your partner ejaculates inside your vagina, releasing millions of sperm that race towards the egg. This is a form of natural selection as it is the strongest and fastest sperm that get there first. Many sperm may be strong enough to reach the egg, but only one will fertilise it. Each sperm swims towards the egg head first. As it reaches the tough outer layer of the egg, it releases enzymes that eat away at this barrier, enabling one of the sperm to penetrate into the innermost part of the egg.

Once inside, the genes of the sperm and egg combine to create a new and unique genetic code, which will determine your baby's physical characteristics (see pages 12–13).

Fit to conceive

You and your partner can improve your fertility by following a healthy lifestyle. Looking after your body will not only boost your chances of conceiving but will also help you to cope with pregnancy, labour – and the demands of looking after a new baby.

Get fit

Regular exercise that raises your heart and breathing rate can make a world of difference. For example, a brisk 30-minute walk, just three times a week, can make you fitter and healthier and improve your mental wellbeing (see pages 28 and 29).

Eat healthily

Opt for a diet that contains lots of fruit and vegetables and is relatively low in fat (see pages 20–23). Choose to include plenty of green leafy vegetables, and take take folic acid supplements, as this can help to prevent some fetal disorders such as spina bifida (which is a malformation

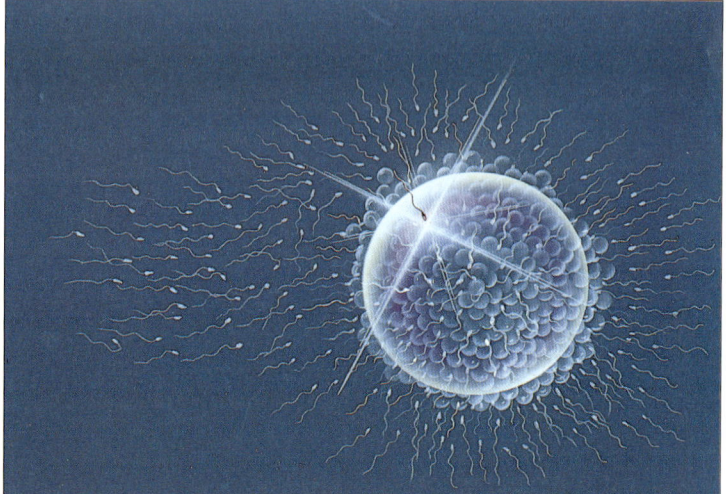

of the baby's spinal column). To boost your intake of vitamins and minerals, avoid overcooking vegetables, as this reduces their nutritional content, and eat lots of raw fruit. All fruit and vegetables must be carefully washed before use to remove pesticide residues and avoid contamination by

harmful micro-organisms. As an added precaution, remove all peel or outer leaves, and scrape root vegetables.

Drink sensibly

Excess alcohol can affect your partner's sperm production. During pregnancy, excess drinking on your part (more than one unit per day) may harm your baby's development (page 24–25).

Stop contraception

If you are taking the contraceptive pill, finish the course before trying to start a family or you may disrupt your hormonal balance. When you come off the pill, wait at least a month before trying for a baby and in the meantime use barrier contraception (such as the diaphragm or condom). If you are using another method, such

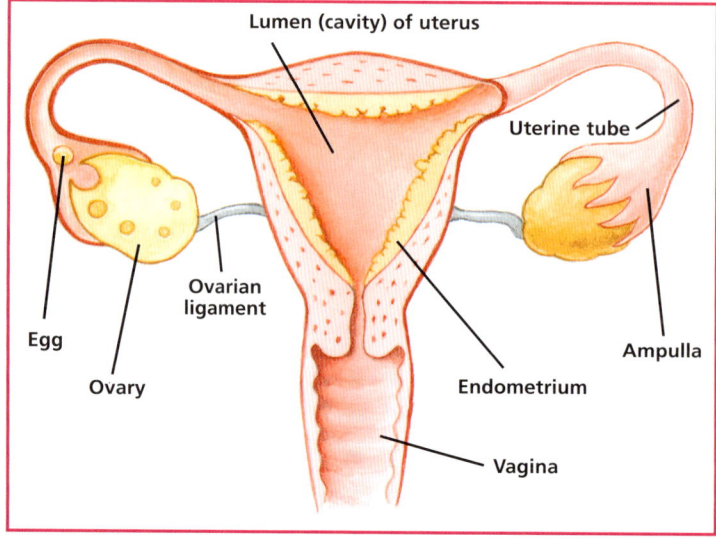

Lumen (cavity) of uterus

Uterine tube

Egg

Ovarian ligament

Ovary

Endometrium

Ampulla

Vagina

Ovaries and uterine tubes.

as the IUCD (or 'coil'), hormonal injection or implant, talk to your doctor or clinic about the best time to start a family.

Time it right

You can become pregnant only around ovulation. This occurs 14 days before the start of the next expected period – around the mid-point of a typical 28-day menstrual cycle. Some women have cycles that are shorter or longer than this, or are irregular. Your egg is viable, on average, for about two days. Sperm can survive inside you for a longer time – around three or four days. Many doctors recommend that couples wishing to start a family should make love regularly for one or two days before ovulation is expected, so that sperm are present and waiting for the egg.

Know your body

You can improve your chances of conceiving by recognising the changes in your body that occur around ovulation. For example, one or two days before ovulation, a watery and stretchy substance called fertile mucus appears in the vagina.

Fertile mucus will support and nourish the sperm, so you can become pregnant any time it is present. Your temperature will rise slightly after ovulation (by up to 1°F or 0.2°C) when taken first thing in the morning using a special fertility thermometer. Some women also experience a dull ache or stabbing pain around ovulation.

By monitoring these changes over several cycles you can work out when you are likely to be at your most fertile. Don't be ruled by the calendar or thermometer, however. All fertility specialists agree that the best way to get pregnant is simply to have plenty of relaxed, unhurried and passionate sex – especially around the mid-point of your menstrual cycle.

WEEK-BY-WEEK

What you do over the next nine months can affect your baby's start in life, so it is important to be as informed as you can. On average, a baby takes around 38 weeks to reach term, or maturity in the womb. However, as it can be difficult to predict when conception actually occurred, doctors usually count term as 40 weeks, taken from the first day of your last period. This means that conception actually occurs around week three.

Over the following pages, 'weekly' panels will chart the progress of your pregnancy over these 40 weeks. Each week, 'What's happening to you' will explain what's going on inside your body, while 'What's happening to your baby' will describe your baby's growth and development.

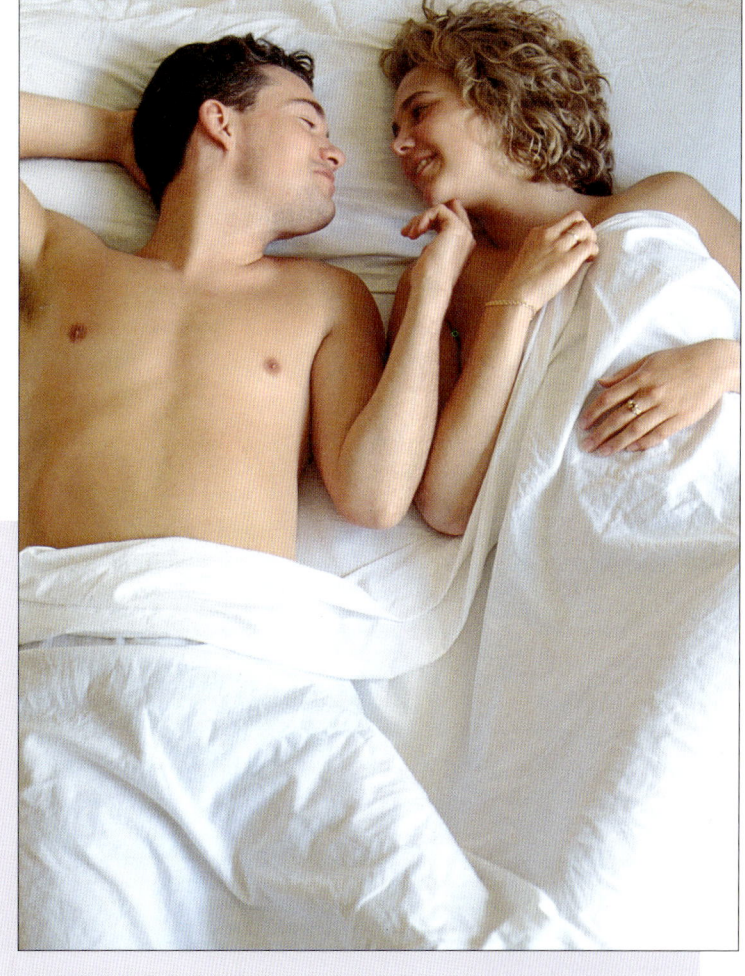

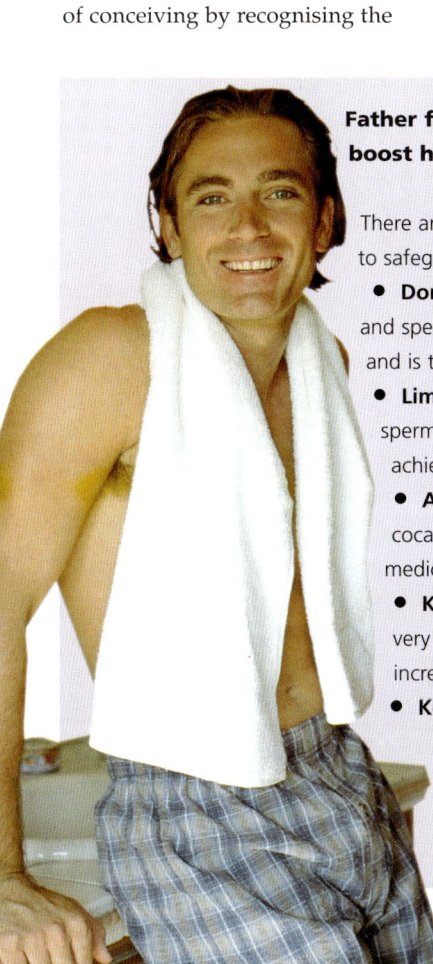

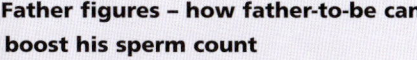
Father figures – how father-to-be can boost his sperm count

There are a few simple steps that men can take to safeguard and improve their fertility.

- **Don't smoke.** Nicotine lowers sperm count and sperm motility (independent movement) and is toxic to sperm in cervical mucus.
- **Limit alcohol.** Heavy drinking can lower sperm count (and impair a man's ability to achieve an erection).
- **Avoid drugs.** Recreational drugs such as cocaine and marijuana and certain medications can affect sperm count. Check with your doctor if you are taking prescription drugs.
- **Keep cool.** Sperm production is affected by high temperature, so be aware of the effect of fever, tight underwear, very hot working environments, a sedentary lifestyle, saunas and hot baths, as they can decrease male fertility by increasing testicular heat.
- **Keep your weight down.** Excess weight can raise temperature with a corresponding decrease in sperm production.
- **Examine your body.** If you detect a scrotal swelling that feels like a bag of worms, see your doctor. It may be a varicocele (a collection of scrotal varicose veins). This requires surgery as it can affect fertility by increasing scrotal temperature.

PREGNANCY DANGERS

IT IS IMPORTANT to protect yourself and your baby against potentially harmful infections. Although the risks are slight, they should not be ignored, especially before conception and during the crucial early weeks of pregnancy. Learning to recognise the dangers and knowing how to avoid them are the best ways of safeguarding your baby.

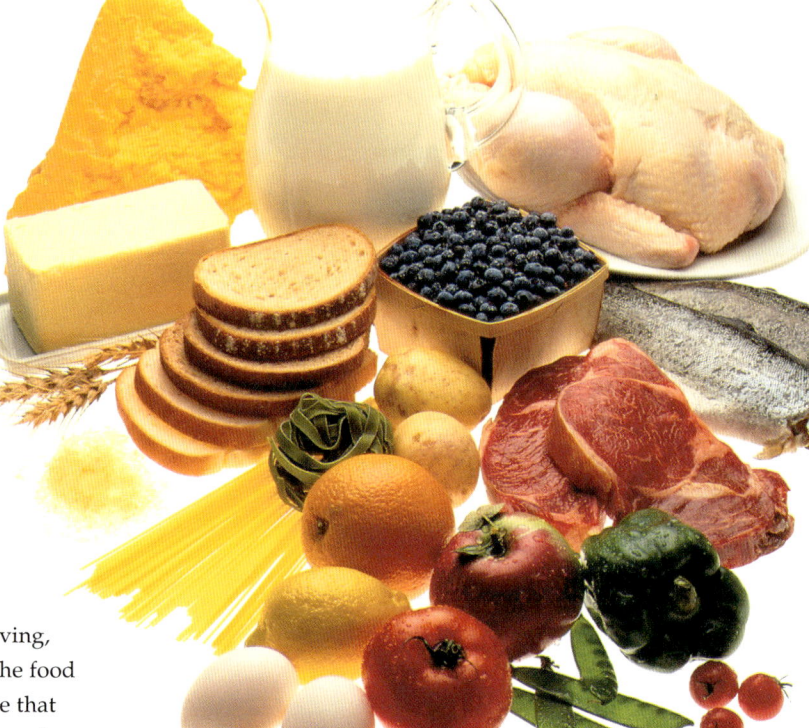

FACT BOX

Food left at room temperature allows bacteria to multiply to levels that may harm you and your baby.

As well as making sure you are getting the right nutrients, you should also be careful to avoid contaminated food. Food poisoning can lead to miscarriage so always follow good hygiene practice. There is a lot of truth in the saying 'keep hot food hot and cold food cold'. In essence, this means don't leave cooked food lying around uncovered, or let refrigerated food get too warm.

Kitchen dangers

The kitchen is a potentially dangerous place, but you can minimise the risks. Take extra care when preparing and storing food and avoid high-risk foods, such as shellfish (especially raw oysters).

STORAGE: Keep cooked food near the top of the refrigerator and raw food near the bottom, or use sealable containers. This

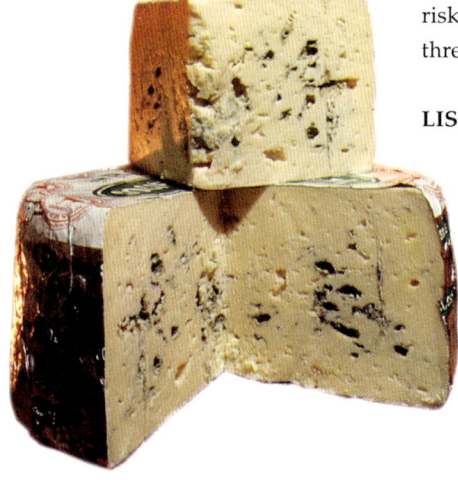

prevents germs from uncooked foodstuffs dripping onto prepared foods.

HYGIENE: Wash your hands thoroughly before preparing food, and use different utensils and work surfaces for preparing cooked and uncooked food.

COOKING: Before serving, check that all parts of the food are piping hot to ensure that any harmful bacteria have been destroyed. This is especially important with re-heated chicken dishes (or better still, avoid reheated chicken dishes altogether).

Special threats

During pregnancy, you and your baby may be vulnerable to risks that would not pose a threat in other circumstances.

LISTERIA: This bacterium is rare, but even a mild infection may result in a termination or severe illness and disability. The risk is greatest in raw and undercooked meat dishes (such as steak tartare, or 'pink' lamb) and foods made with

unpasteurised milk. Avoid the following completely: green top milk (it has not been pasteurised or Ultra Heat Treated), ripened soft cheeses (such as Brie or Camembert); unpasteurised sheep and goat's cheeses, blue-veined cheeses (such as Stilton or Roquefort), and all meat patés.

SALMONELLA: Mothers-to-be are particularly vulnerable to this bacterium which is often found in raw eggs and chicken. Cook eggs thoroughly and

avoid dishes such as hollandaise sauce, meringues and home-made mayonnaise that may have been made with raw eggs. Ensure frozen chicken is defrosted and cooked right through before serving. (Insert a skewer – the juices that run out should be clear.)

TOXOPLASMOSIS: This parasitic condition is caused by an organism found in raw meat, dog and cat faeces and contaminated soil. It is relatively harmless to most adults but if

HIV/AIDS
Testing will help your baby

If you or your partner may have been exposed to HIV, the virus that causes AIDS (acquired immune deficiency syndrome), you should be screened for it before you decide to try for a baby or as early as possible in pregnancy. The virus can be transmitted via the blood, semen or vaginal secretions of an infected person, even if he or she shows no outward signs of the infection.

There is a 15 per cent chance of an HIV-positive mother passing the virus to her baby through the placenta or during birth. Anti-HIV drugs can be taken during pregnancy to reduce the risk of infection, so early detection is important. The risk is halved if delivery is by Caesarean section.

contracted by a pregnant women can cause serious damage to the fetus, including blindness and mental retardation. Make sure meat is cooked right through and wash vegetables thoroughly. Wear rubber gloves when gardening and when cleaning out the litter tray – or get someone else to do it.

VITAMIN A: This vitamin, although vital in moderation, can harm a developing fetus when taken in excess. During pregnancy, avoid vitamin A supplements, fish liver oil, and all forms of liver, whether cooked or in paté form.

Other risks

There are other potential risks which, although minimal, you may wish to reduce further. For example, by avoiding peanuts and foods that contain them during pregnancy you may reduce the risk of your baby developing peanut allergy after he or she is born. This is particularly important if allergies run in your family.

Rubella immunity

Before you try to conceive you should check with your doctor to make sure you are immune to the rubella virus (German measles). If you are already pregnant, a simple blood test in a laboratory will show whether or not you have the antibodies that bestow protection on you and your unborn child. Rubella may cause malformations of the fetus, especially in the early stages of pregnancy, resulting in blindness, deafness or heart disease.

If you think you may have had contact with rubella, don't worry, just talk to your doctor. You can have antibodies in the form of gamma globulin to fight the virus.

Good hygiene, careful treatment of raw meat and avoiding unpasteurised dairy produce are sensible practices if you are pregnant.

WEEKS 1-2

You are trying for a baby and will ovulate at the end of week two. Once the sperm and egg meet and successfully combine deep inside your body, the beginnings of life will be stirring inside you. Many complex developments now start to take place as the first steps along the road to producing a new life.

What's happening to you
- Once the fertilised egg has travelled down the uterine tube and reached the uterus, the pregnancy has begun in earnest.

- Your uterus then begins to enlarge and the walls soften so the fertilised egg, or zygote, can more easily implant in the lining.

What's happening to your baby
- The zygote takes 10 days to travel down the uterine tube and become embedded in the uterus. Its cells are dividing and multiplying the whole time as it does so. At first it is just a ball of cells, which embryologists call a blastocyst. It looks rather like a microscopic blackberry.

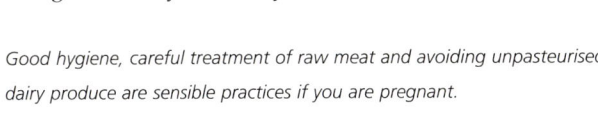

THE LOTTERY OF LIFE

BY THE END of week two, you are at the start of one of nature's most fascinating processes – the creation of a new life. After nine months, what started out as one tiny cell dividing itself into two will have become an incredibly complex infant human, made up of billions of cells.

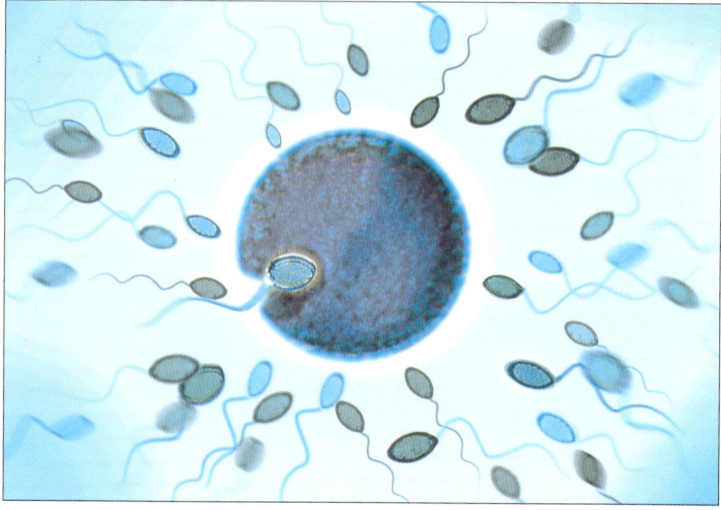

Your baby's genetic code is a unique combination of the genes of you and your partner, which is created when the egg is fertilised.

When a single sperm fertilises one of your eggs, your baby's genetic code is set. Each cell in your body carries your genetic code – the blueprint for every detail that determines how your body looks and functions. A baby's genetic code contains half of the mother's genes and half of the father's. This is because the sex cells – eggs and sperm – only contain half the full complement of genetic material, or chromosomes.

Blueprint for a baby

At conception, the mother's egg cell, which contains 23 chromosomes, and the father's sperm cell, which also contains 23 chromosomes, combine to make a cell that has the full complement of 46. This cell is the starting point, no bigger than a pin head, that will eventually grow into your baby.

Boy or girl

The sex of your baby is determined by the genetic makeup of the sperm that fertilises the egg. One of the 23 chromosomes in both the egg and the sperm holds a 'sex chromosome'. In the egg this is always an 'X' which determines female sexual characteristics. The sperm, however, may contain either an 'X' chromosome, or a 'Y' chromosome, which determines male characteristics.

If the winning sperm (that is, the one that penetrates the egg first) has an 'X' chromosome, the resulting combination is 'XX', a girl. If the sperm's sex chromosome is a 'Y', the result is 'XY', a boy. Statistically, the chances are almost 50/50 – but are slightly tipped in favour of boys, although it is not clear why.

Dominant or recessive

When the chromosomes from the egg and sperm meet they form into pairs. This means that

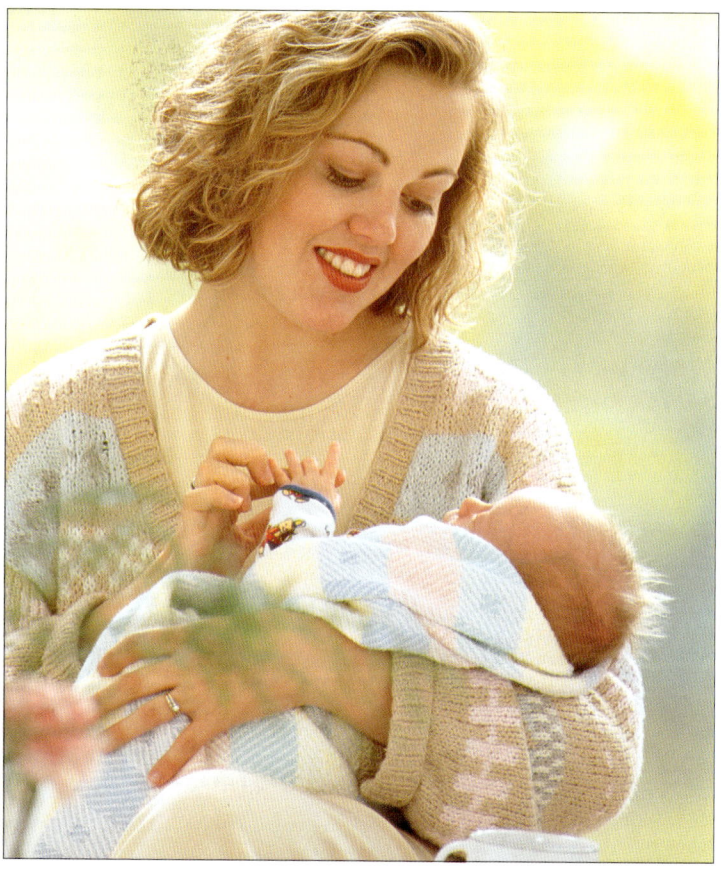

most of the genes they carry are also paired. One of each pair, the 'dominant' gene, takes precedence over the other 'recessive' gene. As a result, there are certain genetic characteristics that are dominant over others, so that you can usually predict the likelihood of your baby having, for example, a particular eye and hair colouring.

Brown eyes and brown hair are dominant characteristics, and take precedence if they pair with, for example, the genes for blue eyes and blonde hair, which are recessive. So, if your baby has two 'brown eyes' genes or a 'brown eyes' gene and a 'blue eyes' gene, your baby will have brown eyes. The baby would need two 'blue eyes' genes to have blue eyes. This is the reason why there are an increasing number of brown-eyed people in the world!

However, even though both parents may have brown eyes, it is still possible to have a blue-eyed baby if both parents carry the recessive 'blue eyes' gene inherited from their parents. Two parents with brown eyes have a one in four chance of having a blue-eyed baby, providing they both carry the recessive 'blue eyes' gene.

MEDICAL ADVICE BY DR. CAROL COOPER

CHOOSING A BOY OR A GIRL

Tipping the scales in your favour

Can you affect the chances of having a boy or a girl? Various authorities believe you can. Their theories are based on the idea that keeping your partner's sperm count high and having sex close to ovulation increases the likelihood of having a boy. Reducing his sperm count, however, and having sex before ovulation favours a girl.

FOR A BOY

- Douche with a dilute baking soda solution.
- Abstain from sex until ovulation or shortly afterwards.
- Have an orgasm.
- Your partner should practise deep penetration during intercourse.
- Your partner should wear loose fitting underwear, drink caffeinated coffee and have a cold shower before intercourse.

FOR A GIRL

- Douche with dilute vinegar and water.
- Have frequent sex shortly after menstruation until shortly before ovulation
- Don't have an orgasm.
- Your partner should practise shallow entry during intercourse.
- Your partner should wear close-fitting underwear, take a hot bath beforehand and avoid caffeinated drinks.

But perhaps we should take all this with a pinch of salt, and let nature take its course!

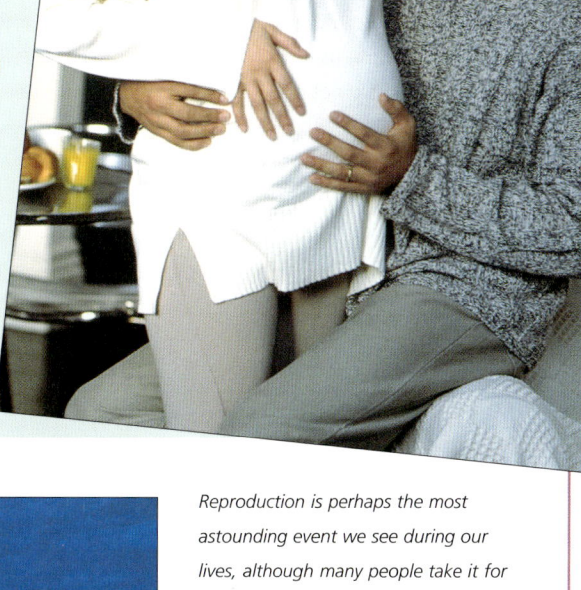

At first unknown to you, there is a tiny miracle developing inside your body. Day by day, what started as one cell becomes more and more complex as it multiplies and grows.

What's happening to you

- You may not feel any symptoms that indicate pregnancy yet – usually the first warning women get will be a missed period.

What's happening to your baby

- The blastocyst floats in the uterine cavity for several days. It secretes a special hormone that enables it to become embedded in the uterine wall (or endometrium).
- Once the blastocyst becomes implanted, some of its outer cells start to form into the placenta. As the placenta develops, it attaches itself to the uterus and acts as a link between you and your baby (see pages 16 and 17). In a few weeks, your baby will begin to take nourishment through it.

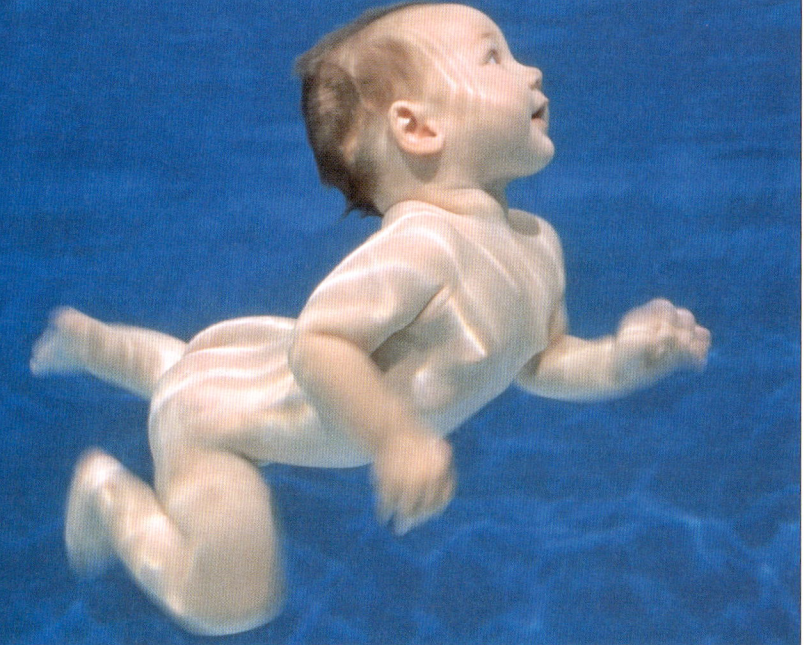

Reproduction is perhaps the most astounding event we see during our lives, although many people take it for granted. It is incredible to think that you and your partner have the power to create another living human being, in all its incredible complexity.

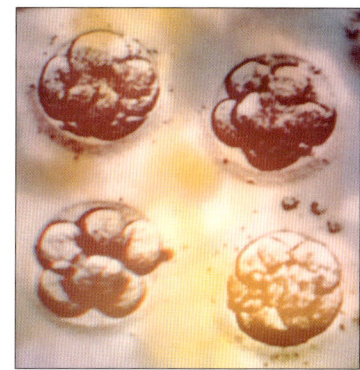

Four day old human embryos in vitro. At first the fertilised egg is just a ball of dividing and multiplying cells which embryologists call a blastocyst.

GREAT EXPECTATIONS

ALTHOUGH CONCEPTION has occurred, it may still be too early for you to be aware of it. If you suspect you may be pregnant, the first step is to visit the local pharmacy where you'll find a range of accurate home testing kits. If the test is positive, the next step is to book an appointment with your doctor.

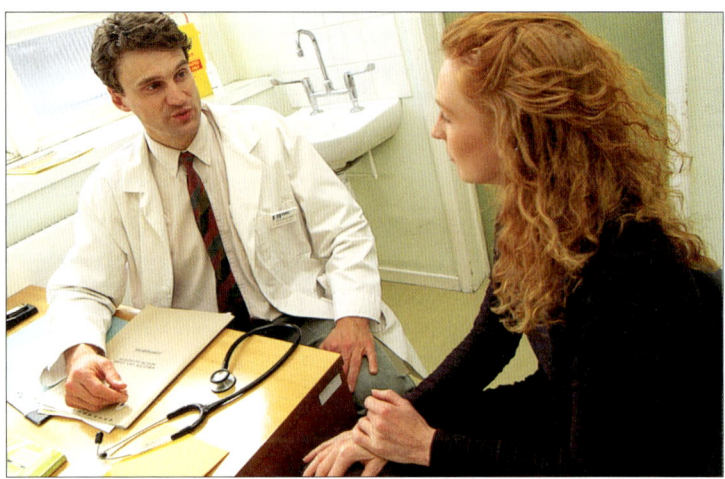

If you think you may be pregnant, don't delay in finding out for sure. The way you look after yourself in the first few weeks and months of pregnancy can have a major impact on your baby's development. While still only a tiny embryo, internal organs such as the heart and lungs are already starting to form – so your baby is particularly vulnerable to damaging substances like tobacco smoke, excess alcohol and drugs.

Testing, testing

There are many pregnancy tests available on the market today. They all work by detecting a hormone in your urine called human chorionic gonadotropin (hCG), which is produced by the developing embryo. The presence of the hormone either changes the colour of a chemical in a test tube or on a dipstick (colour test), or prevents a mixture from coagulating (ring test).

You should perform the test again a few days later even if your period is still late.

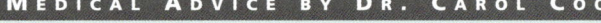
Above: When you first see your doctor, be prepared to answer the questions below.

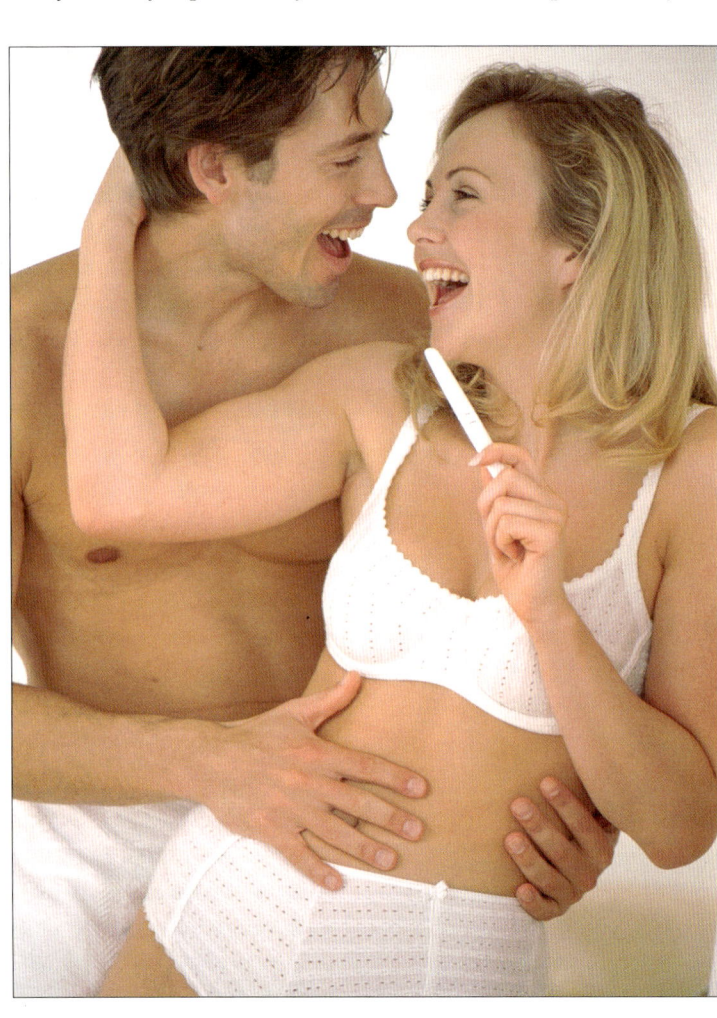

MEDICAL ADVICE BY DR. CAROL COOPER

SEEING YOUR GP
What will your doctor ask?

When you visit your doctor to have your pregnancy confirmed, you may be asked a list of questions. This is routine and does not indicate any special problems in your case.

- You will be asked if you remember the first date of your last period, whether you are pleased to be pregnant and whether you have any fears and worries.
- Your doctor will want to know what happened during a previous pregnancy and labour.
- You will be asked if there is any illness that runs in your family as this may affect your baby.
- Your doctor will want to know if there is anything about your medical history that may be relevant. For example, have you had surgery in the past, or currently take any medication?
- You will be asked about possible drug allergies, whether you smoke and your average weekly alcohol consumption.
- Your doctor will want to ascertain whether you are immune to rubella, have had a cervical smear recently, and are taking folic acid supplements.
- Your doctor will also want to note any preferences you may have regarding hospitals, obstetricians, and type of birth.

Sometimes the first test may be positive, but the follow up test then proves negative. This is because around ten per cent of fertilised eggs do not successfully attach to the wall of the uterus. In that case the first test will detect the fertilised egg, but the second test will show a negative result as hormone levels return to normal.

Testing times

Pregnancy tests work any time from two weeks after conception – around the time of your next period. It is advisable to wait up to four days after your period was due, especially as menstruation can often be late, when the levels of hCG in your urine will definitely be high enough to register a positive result. If you test too early it can give a false negative result. Whenever you test, you should always confirm it by repeating the test a few days later. All kits contain two tests for this reason.

DELIVERY DATE
Calculate the date of the birth

With this chart, you will be able to predict your baby's probable birth date. This will be known as the estimated date of delivery (EDD). Look along the columns of bold figures to find the first day of your last period. The date below it is your EDD.

January	1	2	3	4	5	6	7	8	9	10	11	12	13	14	15	16	17	18	19	20	21	22	23	24	25	26	27	28	29	30	31
October	8	9	10	11	12	13	14	15	16	17	18	19	20	21	22	23	24	25	26	27	28	29	30	31	1	2	3	4	5	6	7
February	1	2	3	4	5	6	7	8	9	10	11	12	13	14	15	16	17	18	19	20	21	22	23	24	25	26	27	28			
November	8	9	10	11	12	13	14	15	16	17	18	19	20	21	22	23	24	25	26	27	28	29	30	1	2	3	4	5			
March	1	2	3	4	5	6	7	8	9	10	11	12	13	14	15	16	17	18	19	20	21	22	23	24	25	26	27	28	29	30	31
December	6	7	8	9	10	11	12	13	14	15	16	17	18	19	20	21	22	23	24	25	26	27	28	29	30	31	1	2	3	4	5
April	1	2	3	4	5	6	7	8	9	10	11	12	13	14	15	16	17	18	19	20	21	22	23	24	25	26	27	28	29	30	
January	6	7	8	9	10	11	12	13	14	15	16	17	18	19	20	21	22	23	24	25	26	27	28	29	30	31	1	2	3	4	
May	1	2	3	4	5	6	7	8	9	10	11	12	13	14	15	16	17	18	19	20	21	22	23	24	25	26	27	28	29	30	31
February	5	6	7	8	9	10	11	12	13	14	15	16	17	18	19	20	21	22	23	24	25	26	27	28	1	2	3	4	5	6	7
June	1	2	3	4	5	6	7	8	9	10	11	12	13	14	15	16	17	18	19	20	21	22	23	24	25	26	27	28	29	30	
March	8	9	10	11	12	13	14	15	16	17	18	19	20	21	22	23	24	25	26	27	28	29	30	31	1	2	3	4	5	6	
July	1	2	3	4	5	6	7	8	9	10	11	12	13	14	15	16	17	18	19	20	21	22	23	24	25	26	27	28	29	30	31
April	7	8	9	10	11	12	13	14	15	16	17	18	19	20	21	22	23	24	25	26	27	28	29	30	1	2	3	4	5	6	7
August	1	2	3	4	5	6	7	8	9	10	11	12	13	14	15	16	17	18	19	20	21	22	23	24	25	26	27	28	29	30	31
May	8	9	10	11	12	13	14	15	16	17	18	19	20	21	22	23	24	25	26	27	28	29	30	31	1	2	3	4	5	6	7
September	1	2	3	4	5	6	7	8	9	10	11	12	13	14	15	16	17	18	19	20	21	22	23	24	25	26	27	28	29	30	
June	8	9	10	11	12	13	14	15	16	17	18	19	20	21	22	23	24	25	26	27	28	29	30	1	2	3	4	5	6	7	
October	1	2	3	4	5	6	7	8	9	10	11	12	13	14	15	16	17	18	19	20	21	22	23	24	25	26	27	28	29	30	31
July	8	9	10	11	12	13	14	15	16	17	18	19	20	21	22	23	24	25	26	27	28	29	30	31	1	2	3	4	5	6	7
November	1	2	3	4	5	6	7	8	9	10	11	12	13	14	15	16	17	18	19	20	21	22	23	24	25	26	27	28	29	30	
August	8	9	10	11	12	13	14	15	16	17	18	19	20	21	22	23	24	25	26	27	28	29	30	31	1	2	3	4	5	6	
December	1	2	3	4	5	6	7	8	9	10	11	12	13	14	15	16	17	18	19	20	21	22	23	24	25	26	27	28	29	30	31
September	7	8	9	10	11	12	13	14	15	16	17	18	19	20	21	22	23	24	25	26	27	28	29	30	1	2	3	4	5	6	7

WEEK 4

By this stage you may be aware of some early signs that can indicate pregnancy. If you've had a baby before, you may remember how you felt at this time, and already suspect that you're pregnant. This can be an anxious time until you have had confirmation. You may also be anxious about your partner – should you tell him now, or wait until you know for sure? If in doubt, buy a pregnancy test, so you can impart the good news with confidence.

What's happening to you
• A mucus plug has formed at the opening to your uterus to protect the fetus. It stays in place until you are ready to deliver.
• You may experience 'spotting' – small amounts of blood, like a very light period. This is a sign that the fertilised egg has successfully attached itself to the uterine wall.
• You may be aware of a strange metallic taste, but most women do not notice any symptoms at this stage.

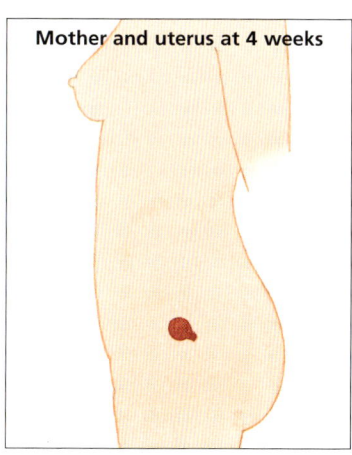

Mother and uterus at 4 weeks

What's happening to your baby
• Your baby's cells are dividing and multiplying at an ever faster rate. From now until the tenth week, the developing baby is called an embryo.
• As the embryo develops, the cells become more specialised for their specific roles. Three layers form in the embryo, like the rings of an onion. The inner layer becomes the lungs, liver, pancreas, bladder, bowels and other internal organs. The middle layer goes on to form the bones, muscles, joints and cartilage. The outer layer will make up the brain, nervous system, hair, skin, nails and teeth.

FACT BOX
Levels of hCG in your urine are highest first thing in the morning, four days after your period was due. For the most reliable result, do the test shortly after getting up in the morning.

BECOMING A MUM

YOU'VE DONE a pregnancy test and it's positive! You are probably finding it difficult to express how you feel – a whole mixture of emotions seem to be rushing through you at once. Now is the time to think about your current lifestyle, and the changes you'll need to make to safeguard your health and that of your baby.

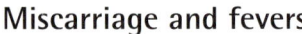

Your feelings are affected greatly by the hormones now pumping round your system. Chiefly, these are oestrogen, which stimulates the uterus to enlarge and helps the milk glands fully develop in your breasts, and progesterone, which prepares the lining of the uterus to accept and nourish the developing baby. Mums who say they are 'feeling hormonal' during the early stages of pregnancy really know what they're talking about.

Early warning

If you only suspect that you are pregnant, it is important to get confirmation as soon as possible – don't put off doing a test or visiting your doctor. During the early weeks of development, your fetus is growing all its organs and limbs, which could be affected by any unhealthy or unsafe actions on your part. In particular, you should look at your lifestyle to make sure you are not doing anything that might harm you or your developing baby.

If you are taking any form of medication, check with your doctor that it is safe to continue. From now on, you must tell all the health professionals you see (including dentists and complementary therapists) that you're pregnant. It may affect the treatment they recommend.

Miscarriage and fevers

More than one in five conceptions result in miscarriage, usually before the tenth week. Many women miscarry without even knowing they were pregnant. Early miscarriages normally show as a heavier than usual period. The causes of early miscarriages are not always known, but many are the result of imperfect embryos that simply stop developing.

Don't take saunas or very hot baths, at least before the 16th week of pregnancy, as this can raise your body temperature and damage your baby. A high fever can also trigger a miscarriage, or harm the baby's development in the early weeks. If you develop a fever try to lower your body temperature by having plenty of cold drinks and taking a cool bath or shower, or sponging yourself down with cold water.

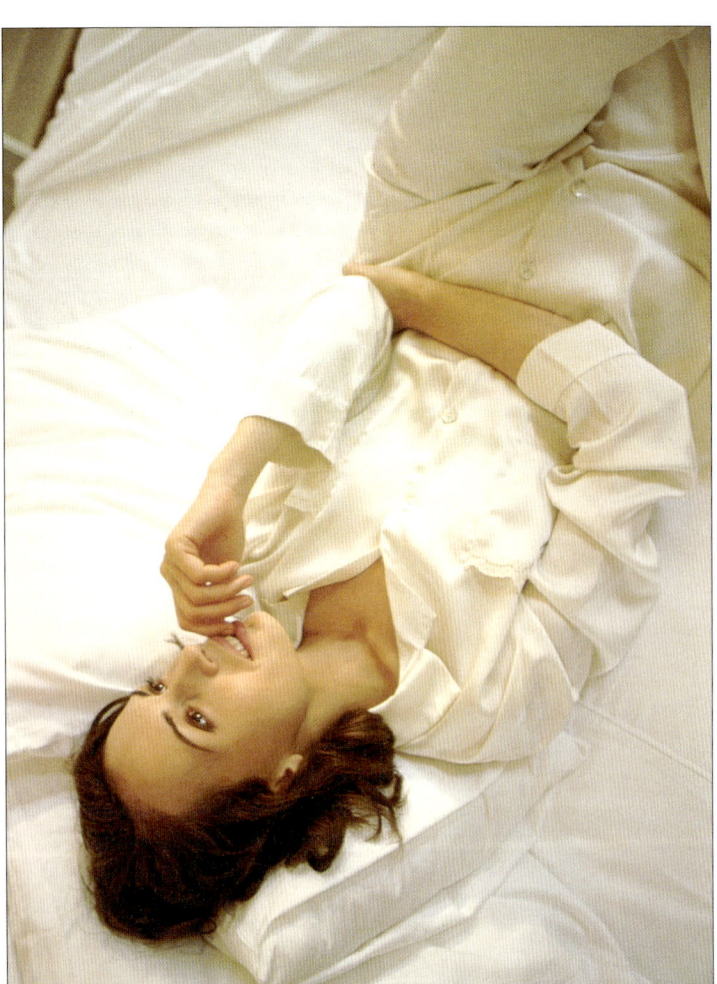

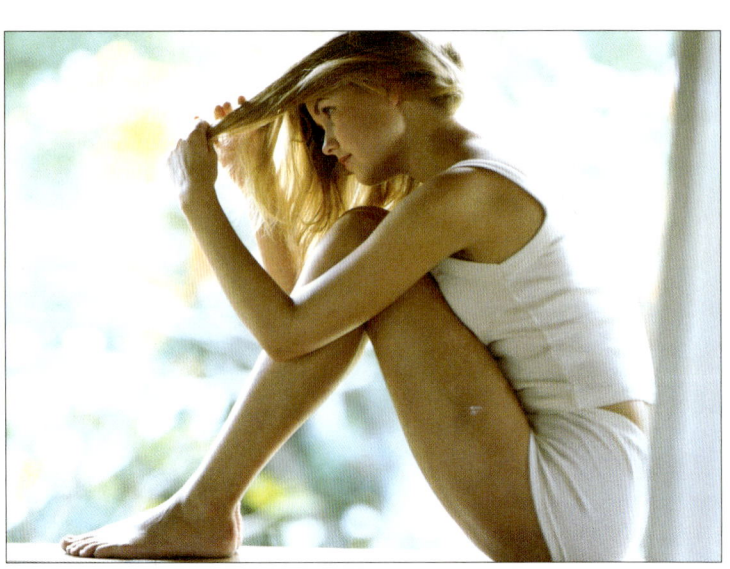

THE PLACENTA

Your baby's go–between

The placenta is a vital organ during pregnancy: it nourishes the baby and removes waste products. Your blood, which is your baby's only source of nourishment, does not go directly into the baby, but is first screened by the placenta, which takes only the nutrients the baby needs. This is why a baby can have a different blood group from the mother, while still drawing nourishment from her.

Your baby does not breathe inside the womb, but takes oxygen, via the placenta, from your blood, and gets rid of waste carbon dioxide at the same time. Not surprisingly, breathlessness is a very common symptom in pregnancy – the heart and lungs have to work even

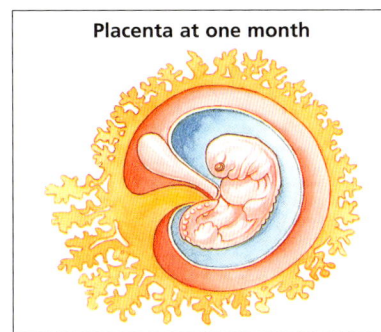

Placenta at one month

harder to ensure that there is enough oxygenated blood for you and your baby. As your pregnancy progresses, the demand for oxygen will increase as your baby gets larger and grows faster, so breathlessness may become more pronounced by the end of the pregnancy.

MEDICAL ADVICE BY DR. CAROL COOPER

TAKING MEDICINES

Ask the experts for advice

Some medicines that a pregnant woman may take can cross the placental barrier and affect her baby. If you are taking medication, tell your doctor that you may be pregnant. If you need an over-the-counter medicine, such as a hay fever remedy, ask your doctor or pharmacist to recommend one.

Never stop taking prescription medication without first consulting your doctor as the baby can be harmed if some conditions are not properly treated or controlled. For example, a severe asthma attack can starve an unborn baby of oxygen. If necessary, talk to a specialist about managing your condition in pregnancy. Although no drug can be said to be entirely risk free, all medicines recommended in pregnancy have been thoroughly tested and are unlikely to cause harm.

It is very important that you seek medical advice about all the medicines you may be taking, even if you think they are harmless. Your unborn baby can be much more affected than you.

WEEK 5

Only when the fertilised egg embeds itself in the wall of the uterus can it be said that conception has successfully occurred. In a minority of cases, the developing embryo may not properly attach, or may find insufficient nourishment for growth. Women prone to this problem may need to take special precautions and may need medical treatment. Talk to your doctor if you are concerned.

What's happening to you
- The pregnancy hormones are now taking control of your body to make sure it develops in all the ways necessary to nurture a baby to term.
- You feel as if your period may be about to start at any moment.
- Your breasts feel more swollen and tender.
- You may feel a little nauseous and may find you need to urinate more than usual.
- Your changing hormone levels may make your skin more greasy, leading to an outbreak of acne. Some women, however, find their skin becomes dry and itchy instead.

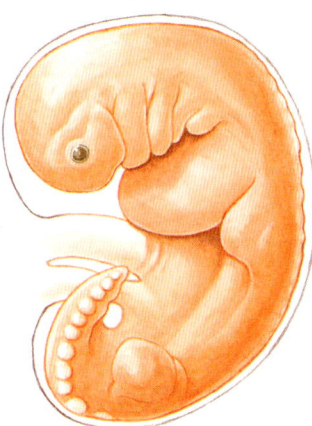

Baby at 5 weeks

What's happening to your baby
- The embryo is 2mm ($^1/_{12}$in) long. It has a head and a tail and the beginnings of a brain.
- A line is appearing along the curved back of the embryo, marking the place where the spinal cord will form. Internal organs, including the digestive tract, are continuing to develop.
- The amniotic sac is developing – this is an envelope of fluid that cushions and protects your baby during the pregnancy. It is this sac that ruptures when your 'waters' break just prior to delivery.

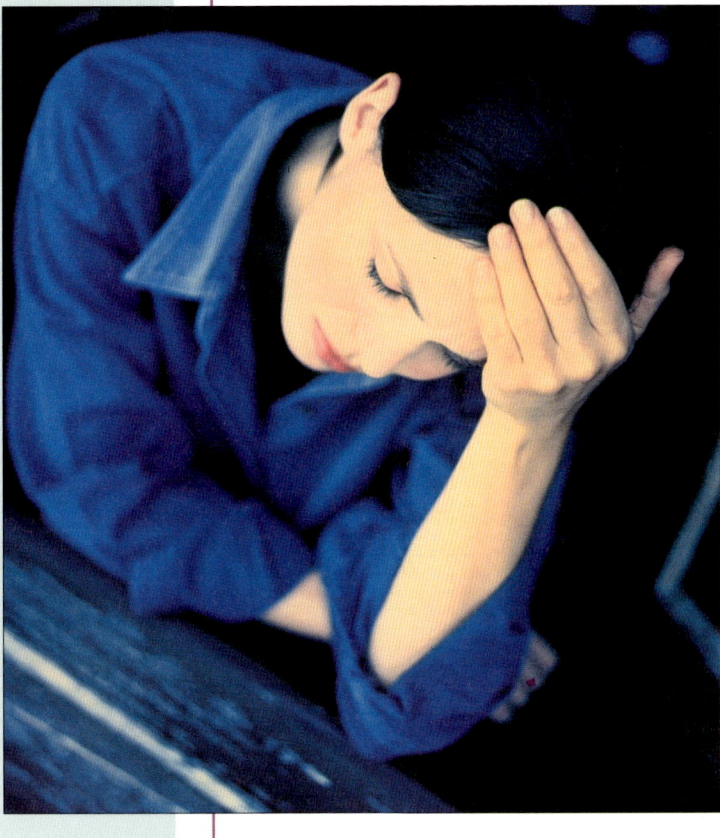

'I FEEL DREADFUL'

MORNING SICKNESS and nausea affect most women during the early stages of pregnancy, and many women say it is the worst aspect of carrying a baby. You may also find you are starting to feel more tired now. But there are steps you can take to minimise or avoid these problems and help you get through the early stages of pregnancy more easily.

Morning sickness is a common symptom of pregnancy and often starts at around the sixth week. Some women may suffer the problem to some degree throughout pregnancy, but in most cases it passes by the 14th week. It is one of the side-effects of the hormones now flooding your system.

Low blood sugar

The problem is often worse when your blood sugar levels are low, so you should eat regularly and avoid missing any meals. Many women find that nausea is worse first thing in the morning,

as this is usually the longest time they go without eating, but it can happen at any time.

A good tip is to eat a cracker or biscuit before you get up. Some women find that sipping a cup of sweet tea really does the trick, whereas others find that ginger settles a queasy stomach. The most important thing is to get something into your system that is easily digested so that your blood sugar levels are raised quickly, letting you return to normal.

Whether morning sickness is making you vomit or you are just feeling queasy, it is important to find time in your daily schedule to take a rest. This is often difficult as others may not know you are pregnant at the moment and so will not be making allowances.

Nevertheless, those who do manage to take things a little easier at this stage often find that nausea is less of a problem.

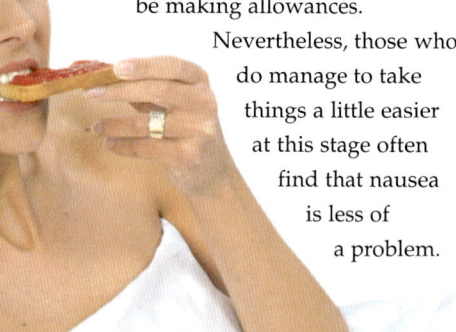

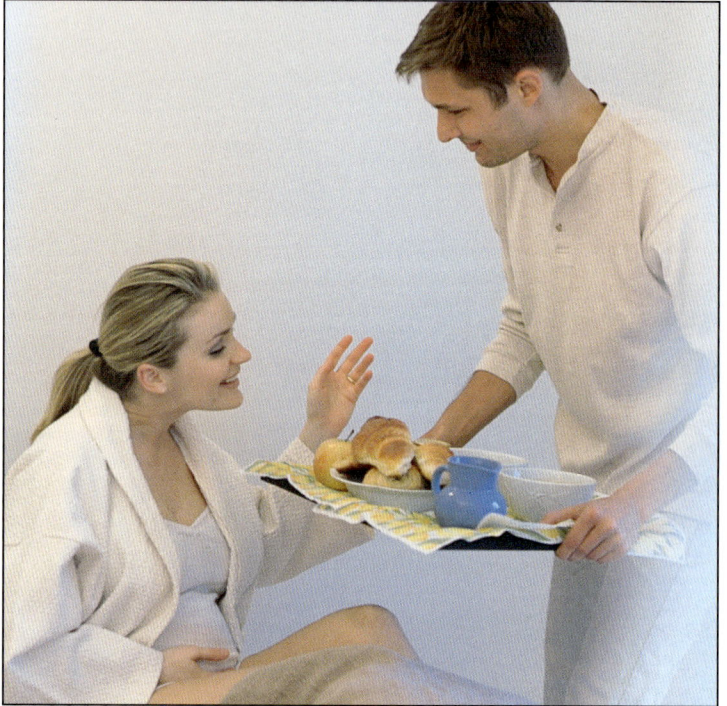

MORNING SICKNESS
Settle Down!

There are some simple measures you can take that may help you to cope with morning sickness.

- Don't rush around too much in the morning. This may be easier said than done, but if possible get your partner to help you with some of the chores, at least during these first few weeks.
- Keep a few biscuits by your bedside to eat before you get out of bed in the morning. When you're feeling queasy you may find ginger biscuits or ginger ale makes you feel better, or try eating a little dry toast, or sucking a mint. Sometimes sipping a cup of hot water can help.
- Eat small amounts regularly and avoid overeating.
- Avoid strong smells, such as spicy cooking or strong perfumes.
- Acupressure bands, used for travel sickness, may be effective. These bands act on acupressure points on the wrist.

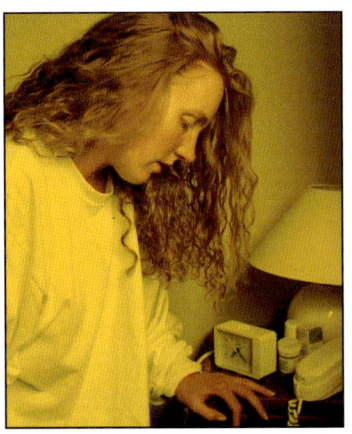

If you're feeling ill and are wondering 'Is it all worth it?' comfort yourself with the knowledge that those who get morning sickness worst are least likely to suffer a miscarriage.

MORNING SICKNESS
When to get medical help

Morning sickness can occur at any time of the day and usually disappears by the end of the first trimester (three months). The cause is not clear but is probably due to a combination of factors. Some doctors think it is due to a hormone acting on a part of the brain that induces queasiness and vomiting.

In order to minimise it, try to avoid rich foods and have a snack or a drink before getting out of bed in the morning. It is helpful to eat or drink small amounts frequently. Pregnancy sickness is rather like travel sickness, so try to move around slowly as this can help.

If the nausea and vomiting is making you feel very miserable, your doctor may prescribe safe anti-sickness medication. Sometimes morning sickness can be very bad, leading to severe dehydration. In such cases, the woman may need to be admitted to hospital for fluids to be administered intravenously (via a tube into the vein). However, the vast majority of women do not suffer the problem to anything like this degree.

Ask your partner to make you a sweet drink before you get out of bed. As well as feeling pampered, this can really help morning sickness.

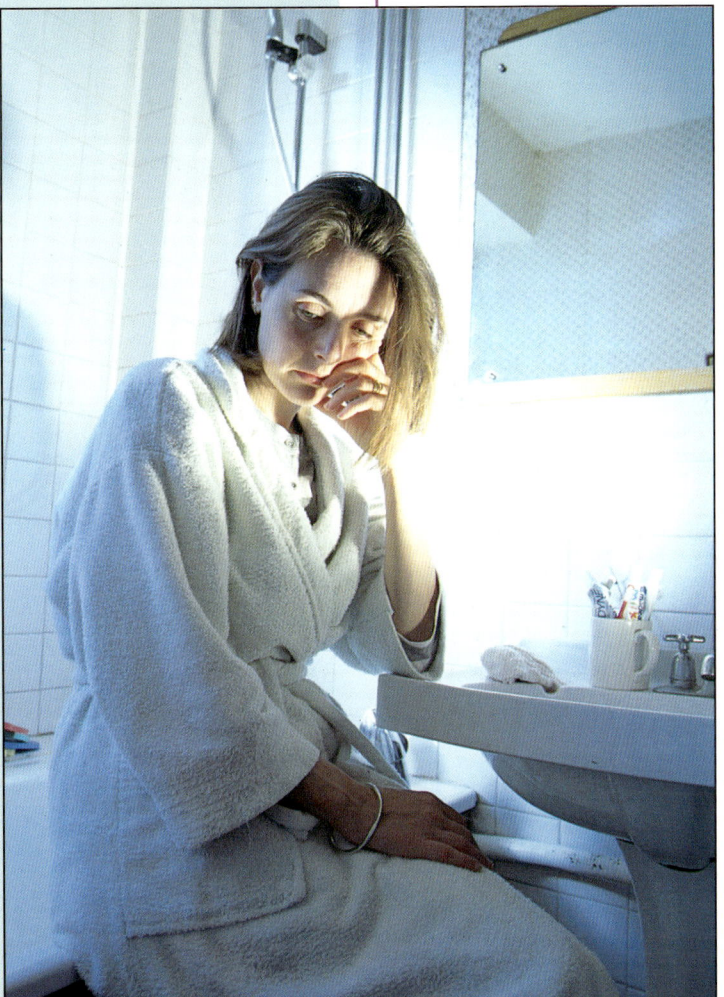

WEEK 6

You are now certain that you are pregnant – you have probably taken a home test and had it confirmed by your doctor. The embryo is now starting to form recognisable physical features.

What's happening to you
- You may be feeling more tired. This is because your metabolism is speeding up in response to the pregnancy hormones. Your body is having to work harder as it adapts for pregnancy.
- You may be experiencing some queasiness, but only about half of all pregnant women have true morning sickness, and of these only one third suffer vomiting as well as nausea.
- You may also notice fluctuating emotions, or mood swings,

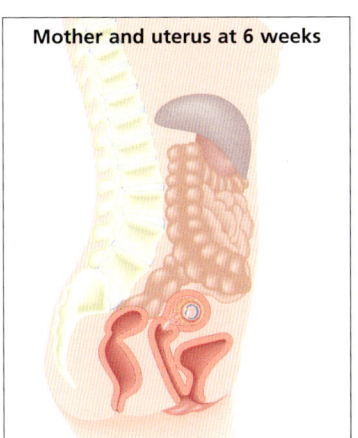

Mother and uterus at 6 weeks

especially when tired, because of changing hormone levels.
- A midwife or doctor is able to confirm pregnancy during an internal examination by feeling the head of your cervix, which has softened.

What's happening to your baby
- The developing embryo is about 5mm ($1/4$in) long and is now shaped somewhat like a tiny seahorse, with a tail, head, torso and limb buds from which the arms and legs will develop.
- Your baby now has the beginnings of a mouth, with ten dental buds starting to appear inside.
- If you were to have an ultrasound scan at this stage, you would be able to see a tiny heart beating, although it only has two chambers rather than the four that will soon develop.
- Blood is circulating to and from the placenta, and there is a digestive system with kidneys and liver. The nervous system is also starting to develop.
- Loops of intestine have formed and are now beginning to receive nourishment from the umbilical cord.

HEALTHY DIET

THE FIRST THREE months are a crucial time in the development of your growing baby and good nutrition is vitally important. By following a healthy diet that provides all the nutrients your baby needs you are giving him or her the best possible start in life. You also reduce the risk of suffering digestive disorders during pregnancy.

FACT BOX

You can increase the amount of iron your body absorbs from vegetables by eating them with foods that are rich in vitamin C.

It is important to eat regularly as well as healthily. Opt for smaller meals, with healthy snacks in between to keep blood sugar levels up, and include a variety of foods to give your baby the widest possible range of vitamin and mineral sources. Plan a diet that is high in fibre, especially from fruit and vegetables, and low in fat. You can increase the fibre in your diet by eating high-fibre breakfast cereals and wholemeal types of rice, pasta and bread.

Try to reduce the amount of refined sugar in the diet. As well as contributing to excess weight, sugary foods and drinks increase the risk of dental problems. Avoid adding extra sugar to food and drinks, and cut down on sweets, sugary snacks and processed foods (which contain high levels of 'hidden' sugar). Your body also now needs extra amounts of certain key nutrients.

Iron

This mineral is vital for making red blood cells. Your baby will rely on the stores of iron obtained from your body until well after birth (up to six months). Ideally, all the iron you need should come from food and is most easily absorbed from animal sources. Iron-rich foods most commonly include meat, oily fish (such as sardines and pilchards), pulses, tofu, green leafy vegetables, apricots, prunes and wheatgerm.

At one time, many doctors prescribed iron supplements for all pregnant women. Now, only those who are shown by a blood test to be deficient in iron are recommended to have them. Excess iron should be avoided as it can cause constipation, a common problem, especially in later months. Women who are most likely to need iron supplements during pregnancy are those who had suffered heavy menstrual bleeding, had given birth shortly before conceiving again (closely spaced pregnancies place heavier demands on the body) or are expecting twins.

Calcium

This mineral is vital for strong teeth and bones. Calcium is particularly important in the later months when the baby's bones become more solid. Good sources include fish eaten with bones (such as tinned salmon and sardines, whitebait and sprats) and dairy foods, such as milk, hard cheese (cheddar) and yoghurt – low-fat types have as much calcium as full-fat types.

As a mother, you will need extra calcium and protein, and milk is a good source of both.

SWEET ENOUGH

Watch your sugar intake

Try to limit the amount of refined sugar in your diet, particularly in hot drinks, colas and sweets, as there is a higher risk of tooth and gum disease during pregnancy. The hormone progesterone causes the gums to thicken and soften, creating gaps around the base of the teeth where food can collect. This encourages bacteria to multiply and increases the risk of dental problems. You can help neutralise harmful bacteria by eating a piece of cheese at the end of meals and chewing sugar-free gum. Brush and floss your teeth diligently and have regular dental check-ups.

The figure in brackets indicates the recommended number of daily servings of each type of food. The size of serving depends on your appetite.

Vital foods	Benefits
Dairy products, such as milk, cheese and yoghurt	Rich in calcium and protein, which are essential for a growing baby. Choose low-fat varieties, which are better for you, but have just as much nutritional value for baby. (2–3)
Fish, eggs, poultry, lean meat, nuts and pulses	Great for protein and other nutrients. (2–3).
Bread, potatoes, rice, pasta	As well as being important energy foods, these are good fibre providers, and so help to prevent constipation, a particular problem in pregnancy. (4–5)
Fresh fruit and vegetables	Rich in fibre, vitamins and minerals. Eat as much as you like of these as they are good for you and your baby. (at least 5–6)

Folic acid (folate)

This vitamin is crucial for the baby's nervous system – deficiency can result in a neural tube defect, such as spina bifida. You should take 0.4 mg (or 400 micrograms) of folic acid every day from the start of your pregnancy; some doctors recommend this as a soon as a woman decides to start a family. You should continue this regime until week 12. There is also evidence that having extra vitamin B12 can reduce the risk of neural tube defects, so consider taking supplements that are specially formulated for pregnant women.

Nutrition is crucial during pregnancy, so try to choose balanced, healthy meals during your entire pregnancy. This is particularly important in the first few months.

WEEK 7

It is important at this time in your pregnancy to rest when you can. If you are usually busy all day, try to cut down on your hectic schedule. You may have bouts of dizziness, especially when standing for a long time. It does not mean that anything is seriously wrong, but is a normal symptom of early pregnancy.

What's happening to you
• You may feel dizzy, in which case sit down and rest for a few minutes until the feeling passes.
• Small lumps may now appear on your areolae (the dark circles surrounding your nipples), indicating the changes occurring as your breasts prepare to produce milk for your baby.

What's happening to your baby
• Your baby is 1.3cm (1/2in) long.
• Your baby has lips, a tongue and openings where the nostrils will form.
• Your baby now has properly developed arms and legs, and small hands and feet have also formed, complete with tiny bumps from which the fingers and toes will grow.
• Your baby's heart is fully formed and is already pumping blood around a tiny, but increasingly complex, network of veins and arteries.

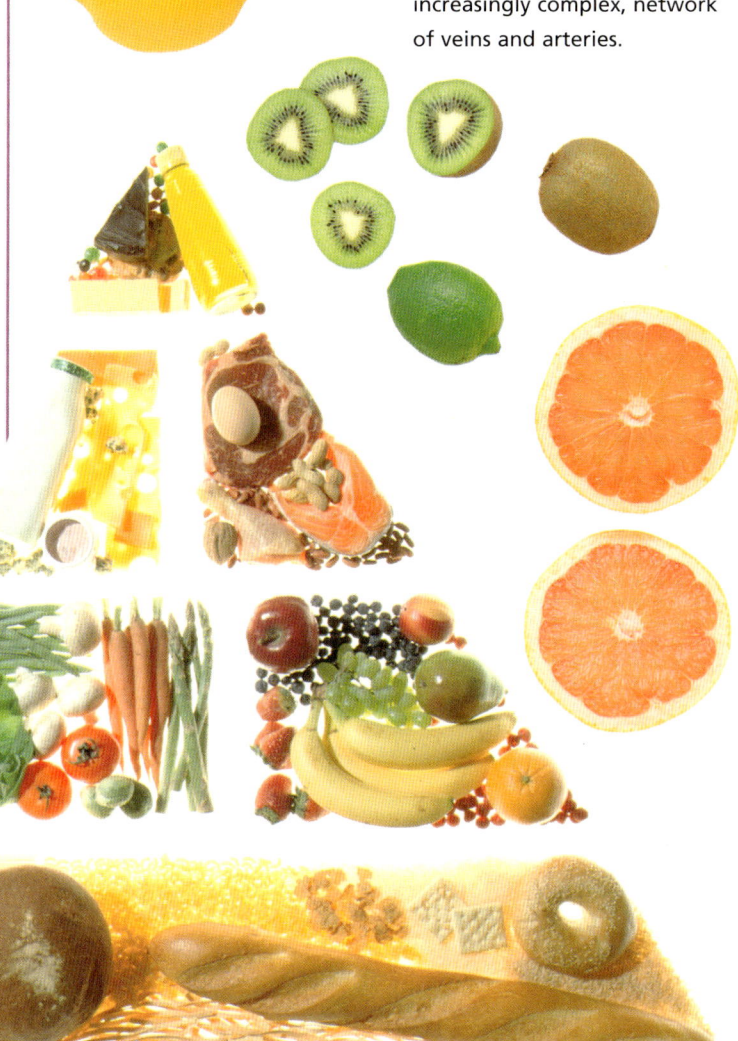

EATING FOR TWO

SOME MOTHERS worry unduly about weight gain as an undesirable consequence of pregnancy. It is far more important to nourish yourself and your baby than to try to control your calorie intake. Most of the extra weight you put on is due to the baby and the changes of pregnancy. You'll soon get your figure back after the birth.

FACT BOX
A craving for non-food items such as coal or toothpaste is called pica. Although harmless it can sometimes indicate a deficiency in the diet.

You must never try to combine pregnancy with a slimming diet. The energy your baby needs for healthy development can only come from the food you eat. If you cut down on the calories you take in it reduces the energy available for your baby to develop properly and to grow to a normal birth weight.

Weight gain

It is normal to put on 9–14kg (20–31lb) during pregnancy. Just because your baby only weighs around 3kg (7lb) at birth it doesn't mean that the rest of the weight you put on is fat. You may retain some extra fluid, especially on your hips and thighs, but the rest of the increase in weight can be accounted for by the placenta, your increased blood volume, the weight of your much larger uterus, your increased breast size, and the amniotic fluid.

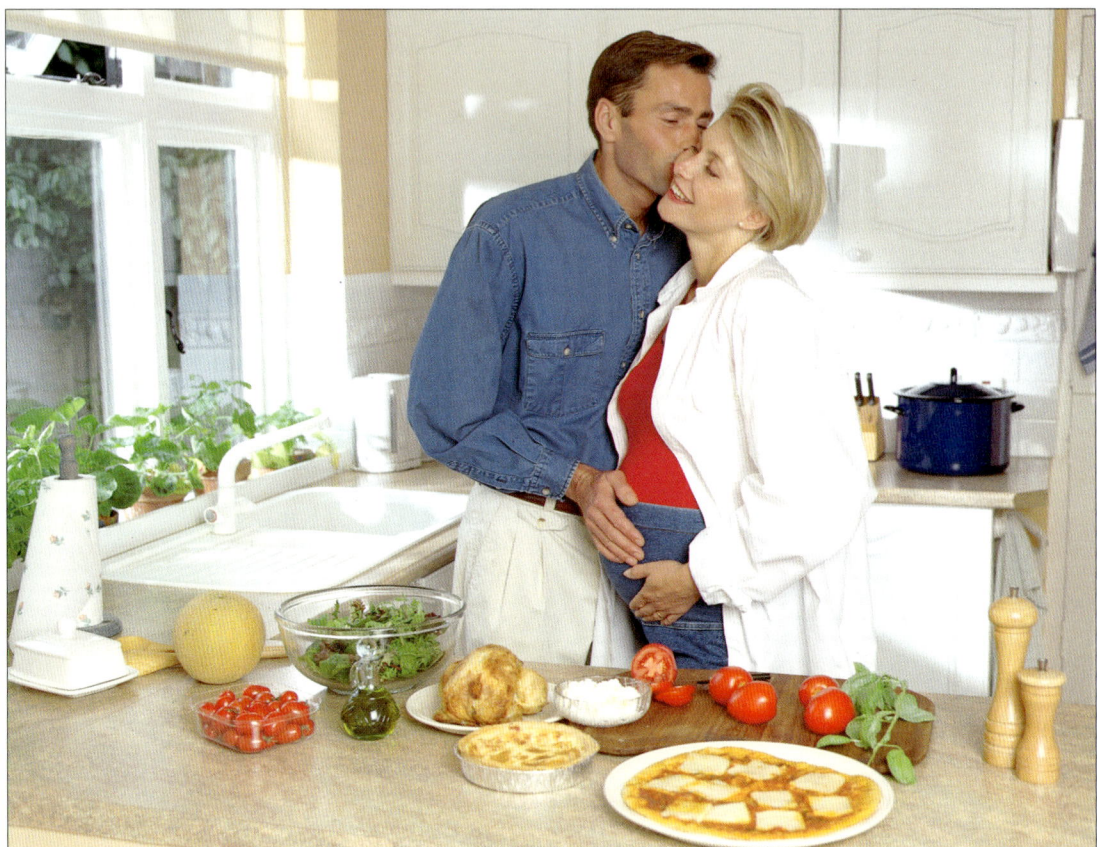

How to 'eat for two'

It is a common myth that you need to eat significantly more during pregnancy. Actually, a pregnant woman only needs to consume an extra 200–300 calories a day in the last three months of her pregnancy (roughly one large jacket potato without butter). The metabolic changes that occur during pregnancy enable your body to use the food you eat much more efficiently. You needn't cut out high-fat and high-sugar foods, such as sweets, pastries, cakes and biscuits, just make them an occasional treat, and not a significant part of your diet.

Fluid retention

Swelling due to fluid retention – a condition called oedema – is a common complaint in pregnancy. It most often affects the fingers, ankles and feet. The best way to reduce the swelling is to put your hands under cold running water and to sit with your feet raised. The swelling is likely to be worse during hot weather and when you have been walking or standing for a long time, or have recently been travelling in an aeroplane.

It is important to remember that drinking less to compensate is not the answer. Cutting down on your fluid intake will not reduce the oedema, but may lead to dehydration, which could cause harm to both you and the baby.

Aim to drink at least 1.5 litres (2¹/₂ pints) of water every day. This includes mineral and spring water, boiled water, herbal teas, fruit juices and squash – but not caffeinated tea, coffee or colas,

Don't feel you suddenly have to eat huge amounts – a pregnant woman only needs an extra 200–300 calories per day.

which increase the rate of fluid loss and cause dehydration.

Although mild oedema is normal at this time, contact your doctor or midwife if the swelling seems to be getting worse, as this might be a sign that your kidneys are not functioning as efficiently as they should. After you have had the baby, your body will quickly revert to normal, prenatal fluid levels.

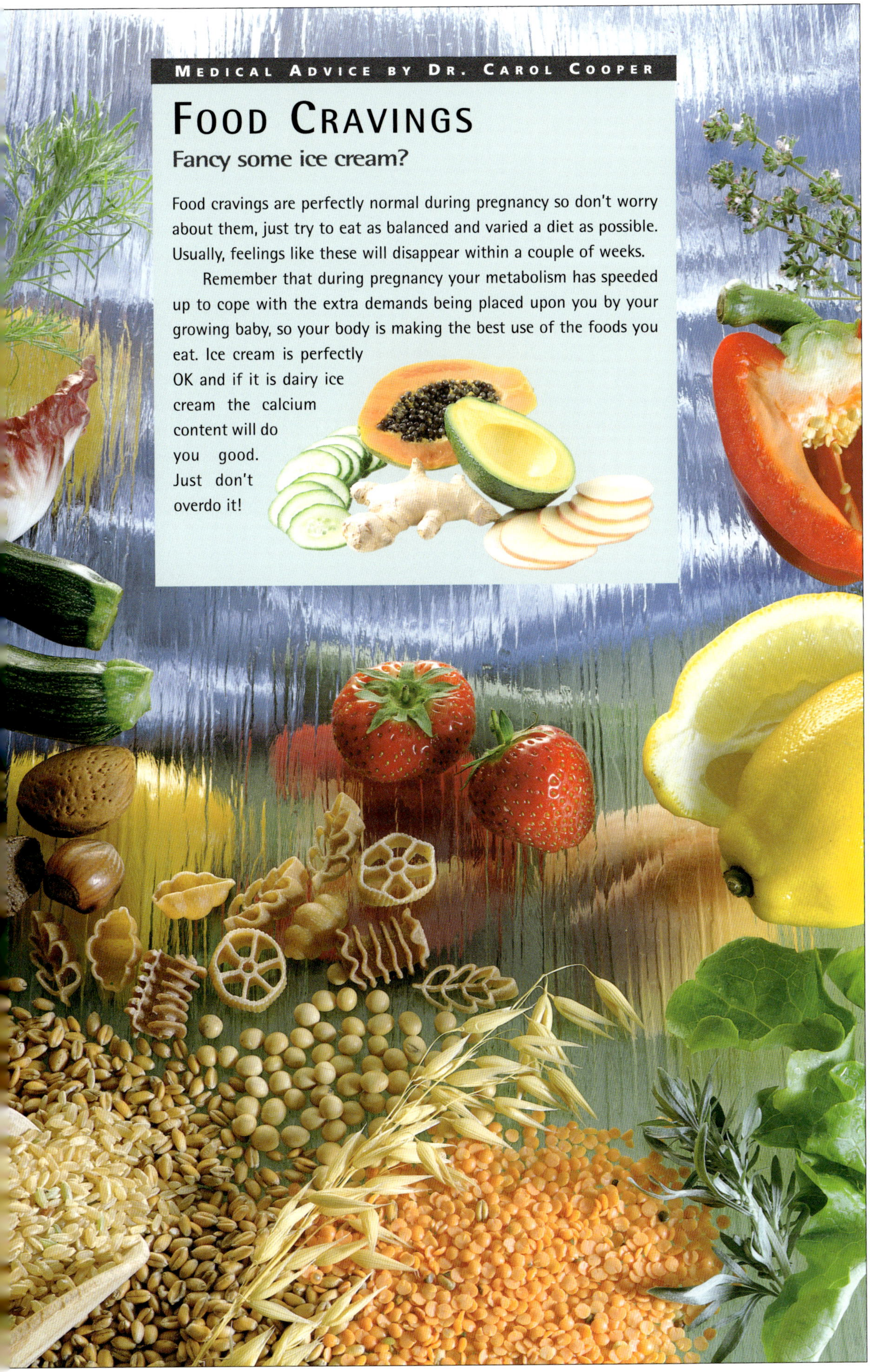

MEDICAL ADVICE BY DR. CAROL COOPER

FOOD CRAVINGS

Fancy some ice cream?

Food cravings are perfectly normal during pregnancy so don't worry about them, just try to eat as balanced and varied a diet as possible. Usually, feelings like these will disappear within a couple of weeks.

Remember that during pregnancy your metabolism has speeded up to cope with the extra demands being placed upon you by your growing baby, so your body is making the best use of the foods you eat. Ice cream is perfectly OK and if it is dairy ice cream the calcium content will do you good. Just don't overdo it!

About now is the time that most mums-to-be start experiencing particular food cravings or aversions, if they are prone to them. Some medical experts believe that these preferences are simply your body's way of registering its nutritional needs. What is certainly true is that your pregnancy hormones affect your senses, particularly your taste and smell. Many women also say they find it easier to give up smoking at this time – if they haven't done so already – and to cut down on other stimulants as the mere thought of cigarettes, coffee and alcohol makes them nauseous.

What's happening to you

• You may be experiencing a slight 'leaking' or discharge from your vagina. If you see any blood, contact your doctor.

• Your hormones are now starting to affect your hair, which may seem drier than usual.

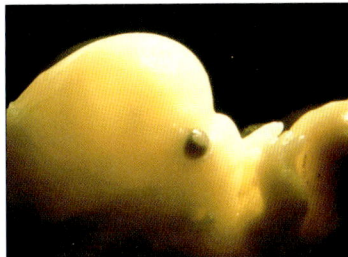

Fetus at 7-8 weeks

What's happening to your baby

• On average, your baby is about 2.5cm (1in) long at this stage and looks less like a little prawn or seahorse, and much more like a tiny baby.

• The eyes and ears are forming, and the face has recognisable features, including the beginnings of eyelids.

• Your baby's main organs are all in place inside the torso and the arms and legs are growing longer every day.

JUST SAY NO!

STIMULANTS HAVE become a regular part of everyday life, whether it's a cup of tea or coffee in the morning, or a cigarette and a glass of wine after the evening meal. Once you become pregnant, however, you have to consider your use of these indulgences very carefully because they can affect your developing baby.

FACT BOX
One unit of alcohol is equivalent to half a pint of beer, one glass of wine, a small glass of sherry or one 'bar unit' (25ml) of spirits.

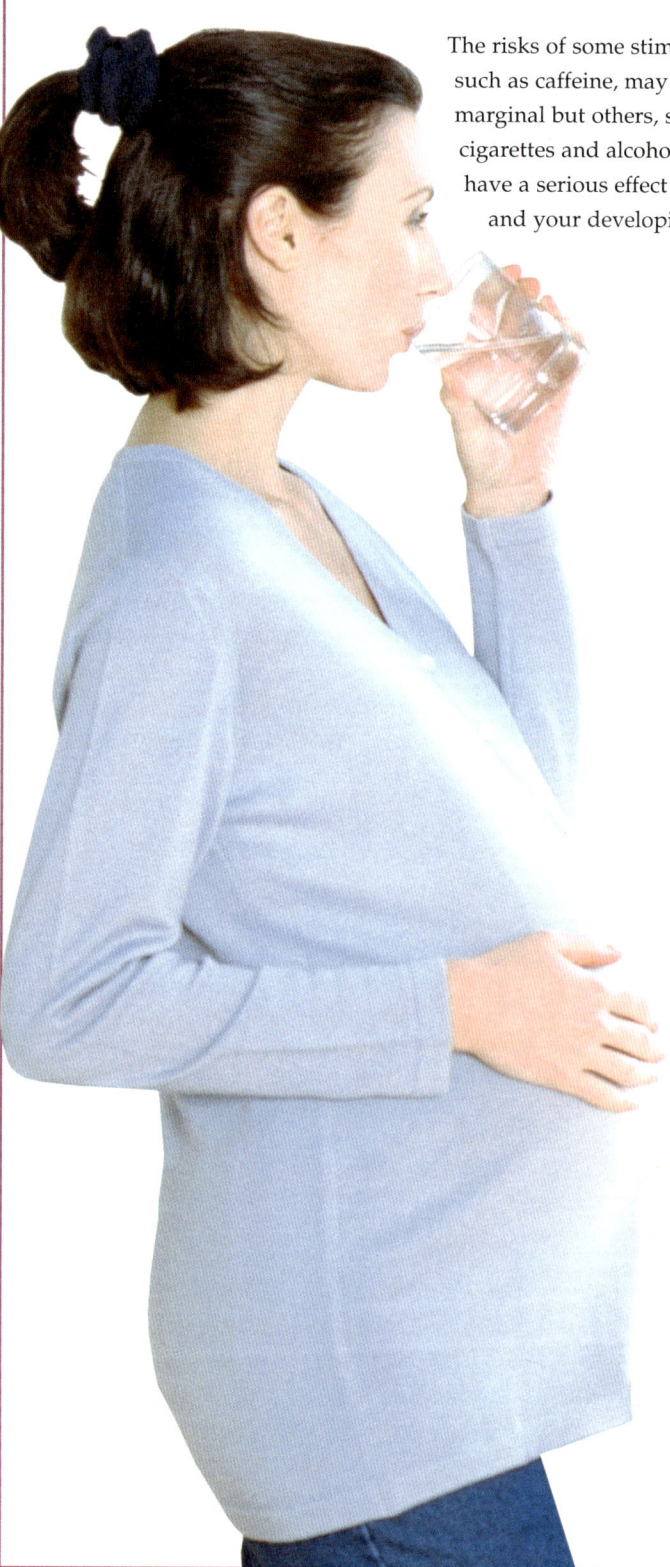

The risks of some stimulants, such as caffeine, may be marginal but others, such as cigarettes and alcohol, can have a serious effect on you and your developing baby.

Cigarettes

Smoking is one of the worst things you can do to your baby. Studies have proven time and again that mothers who smoke have a greater risk of miscarriage and produce under-weight babies. But the ill-effects do not end there. A baby who is exposed to nicotine in the womb is:

• twice as likely to be born premature and under weight;

• more likely to be abnormal in some way;

• more likely to be a victim of cot death during infancy.

Cigarettes produce carbon monoxide, a poison that reduces the amount of oxygen entering your bloodstream. This means that less oxygen is reaching the baby through the placenta, thus causing the baby's growth to be restricted. Other chemicals in cigarette smoke, such as nicotine, destroy some of the vital nutrients in the mother's blood so that less of the essential vitamins and minerals reach the baby.

Giving up smoking is really about will power. If you can't do it for yourself, then do it for your baby. Remember that your body's physical cravings will only last for two weeks

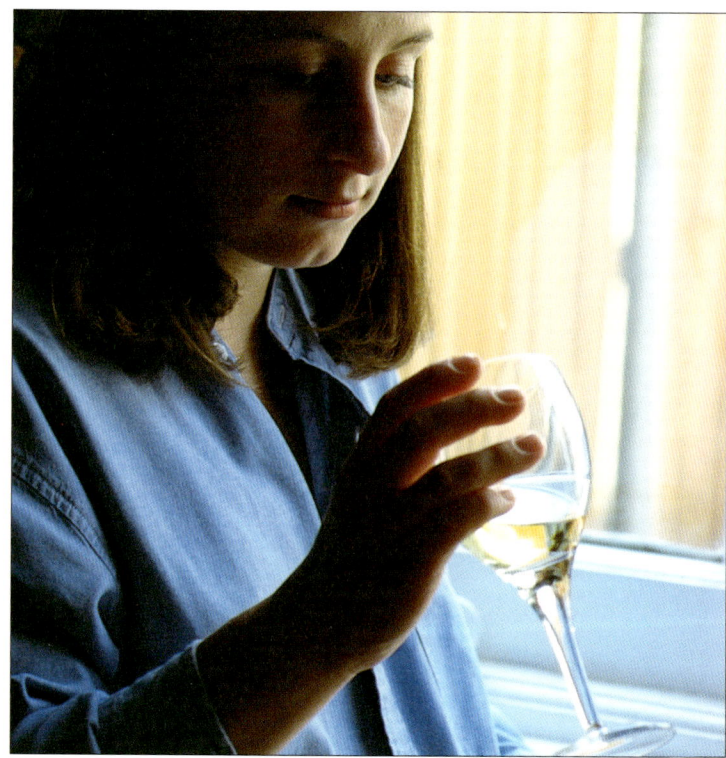

Too much alcohol can have a serious effect on an unborn baby. To be on the safe side, keep to the limits described here (right).

SMOKING
Beating the habit

Hopefully, you will have tackled this very important issue before you conceive. For a variety of reasons, smoking is extremely bad in pregnancy and if you can't quit you should at least try to cut down as much as possible.

Start by throwing out all tobacco products and practise saying 'no thanks, I don't smoke'. Enlist the help of non-smoking friends for moral support. Put your cigarette money into a savings account and watch it grow. Avoid the temptation of smoky pubs and clubs as passive smoking is also harmful for your baby. Congratulate yourself with each week you remain a non-smoker and remember that giving up smoking really will improve your baby's health.

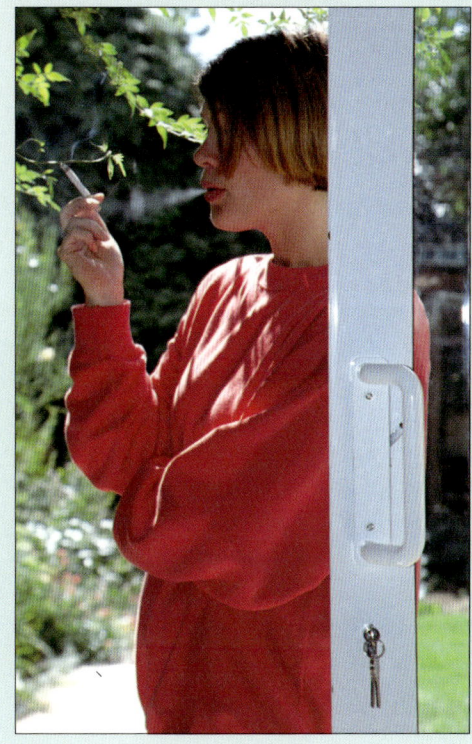

Smoking poses a serious danger for unborn babies. It just isn't worth the risk.

(although it may feel a lot longer for a hardened smoker), and after this period of detoxifying all your cravings are mental rather than physical.

If you're a non-smoker, take care to avoid smoky environments. You have a right to work in clean air, so if smoking is still allowed in your workplace ask your boss to reconsider the company's policy, or ask to be moved to a smoke-free area. If your partner or other members of the household smoke, encourage them to give up or confine their habit to outdoors. If you have to be in a smoky environment sometimes, increasing your intake of vitamins C and E and zinc can help offset some of the effects smoking has on your baby's nutrient intake.

Alcohol

Many women choose to abstain from alcohol during pregnancy. However, provided you are careful to limit your intake to no more than one unit per day, alcohol is not generally considered to pose a serious risk to the baby. Higher levels of consumption may cause problems, however. The type of drink does not matter – it is the amount of alcohol that is crucial (see Fact Box).

If you drink between two and six units per day, your baby has a higher risk of developing fetal alcohol syndrome. This can result in slower growth rate, sight and hearing problems, learning difficulties, and a higher risk of physical abnormalities, such as cleft palate. For every 50 women who drink up to six units per day during pregnancy, up to 12 babies will be born with some or all of these problems.

CAFFEINE
A healthy stimulant?

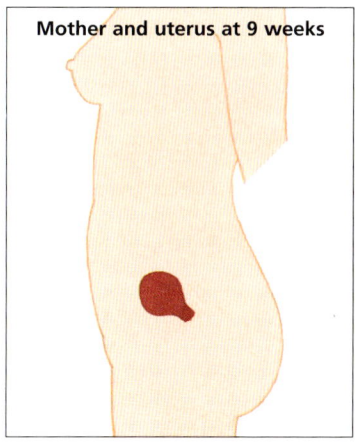

Many experts recommend reducing – or even avoiding – caffeine during pregnancy. There is some evidence that high caffeine consumption may be linked to an increased risk of miscarriage, premature labour, low birth weight, and breathing disorders in newborn babies. As well as tea and coffee, caffeine is found in chocolate, some colas and 200 other foods, drinks and drugs. If you want to cut down on caffeine, check food labels and medication containers to see if caffeine is listed, and look for caffeine-free alternatives. There are decaffeinated teas and coffees available, as well as caffeine-free herbal teas (pictured above) and colas.

WEEK 9

Your skin starts to 'glow' at about this time during your pregnancy, because of the hormones circulating in your system – this is where we get the phrase 'looking in the pink'.

Mother and uterus at 9 weeks

What's happening to you
• You are looking healthier, and friends and family may be remarking upon your blossoming appearance – perhaps the more astute have guessed that you're pregnant, even if you haven't told them yet.
• You will also notice that your waistline is starting to disappear, so you may now be finding your clothes are getting a bit tight. Wear unrestrictive clothing as much as possible.

What's happening to your baby
• Your baby's fingers and toes are really growing now, the hands and feet are looking more like that of a baby, and the wrists and ankles are starting to appear.
• Your baby is also starting to make use of its developing muscles and bones by moving around in the uterus, although the baby is so small (about the size of a strawberry) and the movements so gentle that you will not be able to feel anything.

BREAST CARE

YOUR BREASTS enlarge during pregnancy as they prepare for the role of feeding your baby once he or she is born. In effect, the job the placenta has been doing during pregnancy will be taken over by your breasts after the birth. As your breasts become heavier they will need extra support and care.

Your breasts may now be feeling tender – one of the first signs that you are pregnant. Your nipples are darker and small lumps (called Montgomery's tubercles) may have formed on the areolae. Your breasts will continue to feel tender as your pregnancy progresses, often accompanied by a tingling sensation in the nipples. This tenderness is likely to get more acute as you approach the end of your pregnancy. Your breasts will also feel very heavy and swollen – this is also perfectly normal.

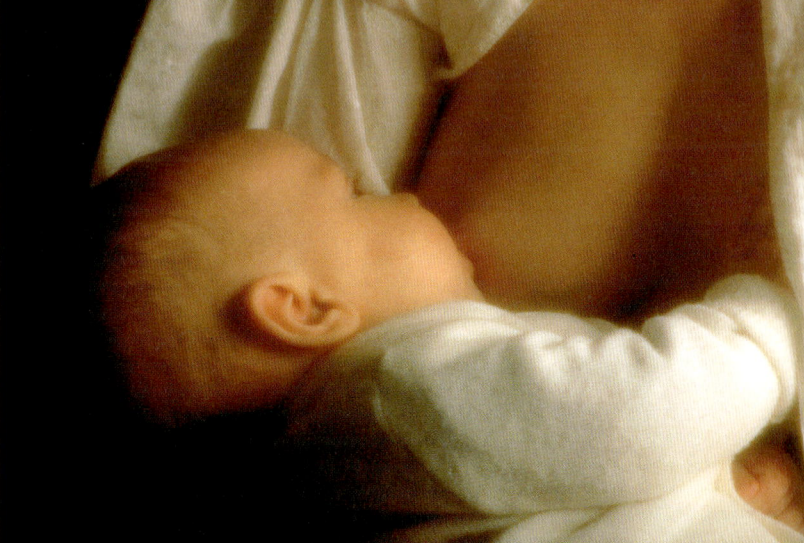

Your milk ducts are developing the role they were intended for, and stretching as they begin to fill with milk.

Supporting role

There is no muscle in your breasts, their weight is supported by a network of non-elastic ligaments which can stretch if too much weight is placed on them. So even at this relatively early stage in pregnancy it is important to find a bra that can support your breasts as they get bigger and heavier. This will go a long way towards reducing the 'sagging effect' of motherhood.

A good maternity bra is one that gives excellent support by having a broad band underneath the cups and wider than usual shoulder straps so that, with the extra strain, they don't cut into your shoulders. It is very important that the back width is adjustable – you will need this in later stages of your pregnancy as your ribs expand to accommodate your enlarging uterus and your back gets broader to cope with the extra weight you are carrying. You may find you need to buy extra bras with a bigger cup size as your pregnancy continues into the later stages.

You should now consider wearing a support bra most of the time during the day and especially when playing sport or exercising, when your breasts are under increased strain. If you have large breasts (size 'D' or larger), it is a good idea to wear your maternity bra at night as well.

SHOP FITTING

Getting the right support bra

You should look for a bra that is snug enough to be supportive, but not so tight that the straps restrict your blood flow. Make sure you get good, impartial advice from those who serve you. Most good stores have specially trained fitters who can help you select the right bra for your needs.

As comfort is your priority, choose a back-fastening rather than front-fastening type. You won't need a front-fastening or zip-cup version – known as a feeding bra – until you are about to start breastfeeding. Feeding bras are supportive and comfortable like maternity bras, but allow you to breastfeed without undoing your bra straps, which can be very helpful when you are outdoors.

Bra manufacturers now produce a range of styles of both maternity and feeding bras. These are available in high street stores, and there are also specialist outlets that supply by mail order. You can usually get more up-to-date information on suppliers from your local parenting group or maternity hospital.

Feeding bras allow you to feed your baby without undoing your bra straps, like this 'drop-cup' version on the right.

> **FACT BOX**
> By week ten, doctors refer to your baby as a fetus (which means offspring) rather than an embryo.

WEEK 10

You are experiencing the breast changes that all mums go through during pregnancy as your body prepares to take on the role of feeding your baby after the birth.

What's happening to you
• You will definitely notice that your breasts are getting bigger and may be feeling tender, especially around the nipples.
• If you are quite fair-skinned, you may become aware of the network of blood vessels criss-crossing your breasts – this can be very noticeable. These are further signs that your body is developing into its maternal role.

• Your uterus is now roughly the size of a small grapefruit, but you won't be able to feel it yet because it is still hidden away behind your pelvic bone.

What's happening to your baby
• Your baby is about 4.5cm (1½–2in) long, and about the size of an apricot. The tiny delicate bones in the ankles and wrists have formed, and the fingers and toes are visible on ultrasound.
• The placenta now starts taking hormonal control of the pregnancy. Until around the tenth to 14th week, one of its hormonal functions has been carried out by the corpus luteum, an area of tissue that forms on the ovary after ovulation. This tissue remains in the ovary and secretes progesterone to support the pregnancy, until the placenta is ready to take over. The placenta releases steadily increasing levels of progesterone into your bloodstream until, by the 14th week, it is in sole command.

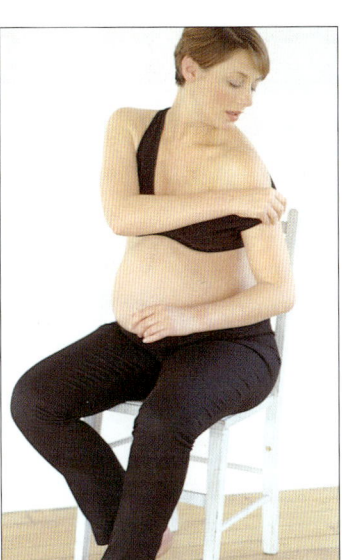

When choosing a bra, it is really worthwhile taking your time.

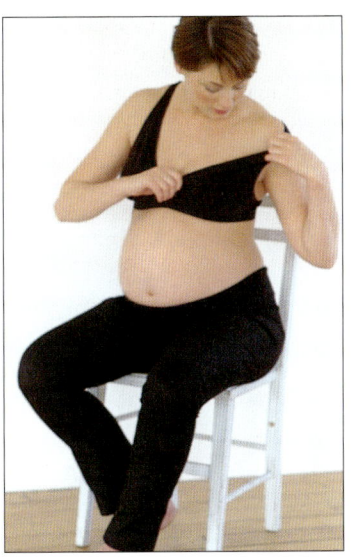

The material should be soft and it should be comfortable for your size.

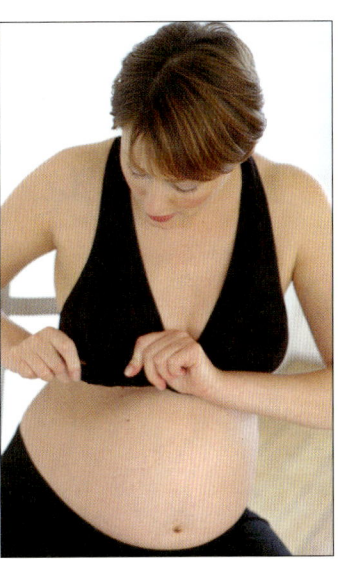

The cups should support without being restrictive, which can affect blood flow.

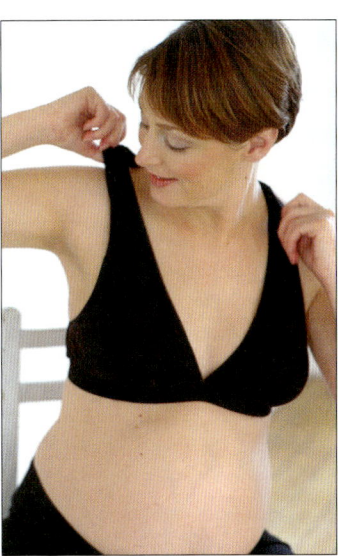

Make sure the straps are wide and comfortable to support the extra weight.

EXERCISE – PART 1

REGULAR EXERCISE can play an important part in keeping you fit and healthy during pregnancy. It can help your body maintain its tone and suppleness and your improved fitness will pay dividends during labour and postnatal recovery. If you are unused to exercising, however, keep to a moderate level of exercise and take care not to overdo it.

The thought of incorporating an exercise programme into your busy daily schedule may not be very appealing – especially if you are suffering some of the symptoms that many women feel during a normal pregnancy. But the exercises suggested here are simple, gentle and effective, and can be done at any time of day with minimum disruption to your daily routine.

Gentle benefits

Ideally, you should get fit before you get pregnant and then maintain this fitness. Alternatively, enrol in a prenatal exercise class. The most important thing to remember is to take it gently – this is not a time to start a rigorous fitness programme, especially if you were not used to exercise before your pregnancy.

Limber up

When exercising, always start with a five-minute warm-up and stretch session. This helps increase blood flow to the muscles and limbers up the joints, thereby reducing the risk of strains, sprains and post-exercise aching.

The simplest warm-up is just to walk around for a few minutes, then repeat the following exercises around six times each. Stop if you feel any pain or discomfort.

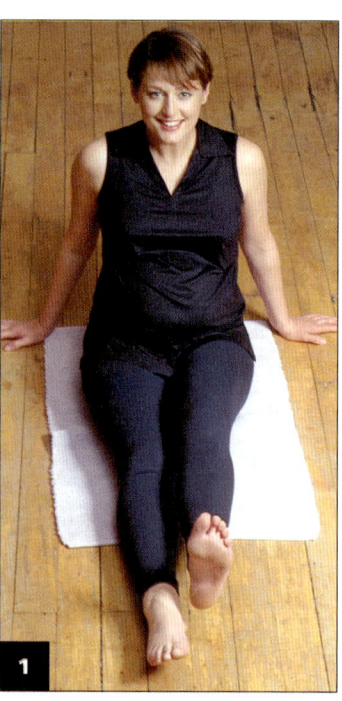

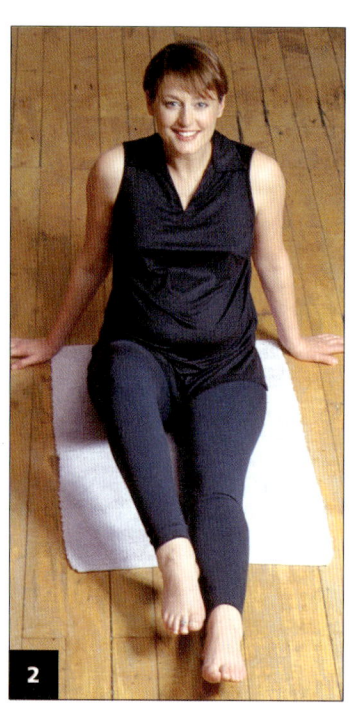

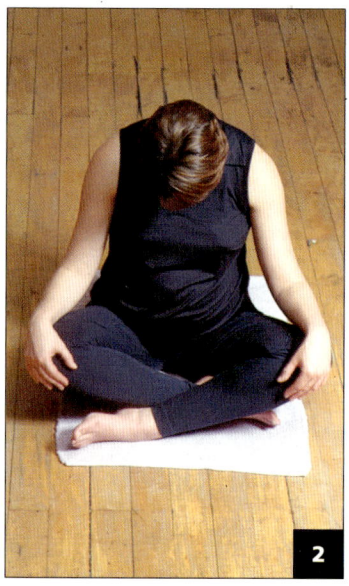

Legs

1. Sit on the floor with your back straight, hands flat on the floor and legs straight in front of you. Bend and straighten each knee in turn.
2. Now raise one leg off the floor and move the foot in slow circles for 15 seconds, flexing your ankle as you do so. Repeat with the other leg.

Torso and neck

1. Sit cross-legged and stretch your neck upwards. Gently twisting from the waist, slowly turn to look behind you, placing one hand on the floor behind you for support. Repeat for the other side.
2. Facing front, slowly lower your head until your chin is almost touching your chest, and then raise it again.
3. Gently tilt your head to one side and then straighten. Repeat for the other side. Always exercise the head and neck slowly and gently to avoid injury.

EXERCISE SAFETY
Better safe than sorry

Ask your doctor's advice before starting a fitness programme as there may be special circumstances in your case that make exercise inadvisable. For example, if a woman has previously suffered a miscarriage some doctors advise against exercise during the first three months of pregnancy. Always follow basic safety rules when exercising, whether you are pregnant or not.

- Avoid jarring or jumping movements as the tendons and ligaments are more prone to injury during pregnancy.
- If you have been a regular exerciser, reduce the intensity of your routine to 70 per cent of pre-pregnancy levels and regularly monitor your heart rate.
- Don't overheat. Aerobic exercise, such as brisk walking, jogging, cycling and step aerobics, quickly raises body temperature.
- Drink water before, during and after exercise to avoid dehydration. A little at a time is best.
- Wear a good support bra (see pages 26 and 27).
- Stop immediately if you feel discomfort or pain, breathlessness or dizziness. If pain persists for more than a day, see your doctor.

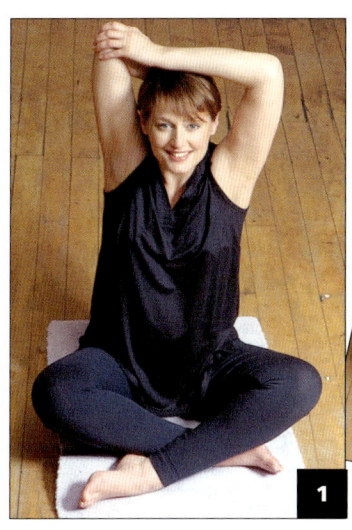

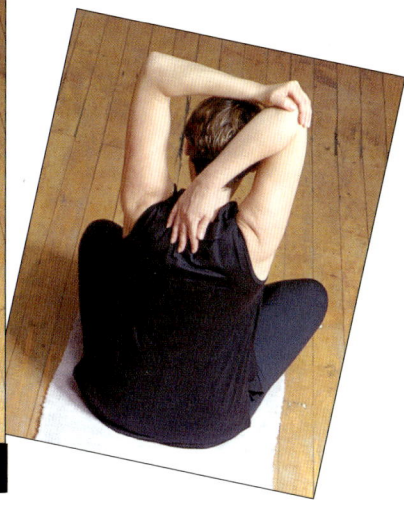

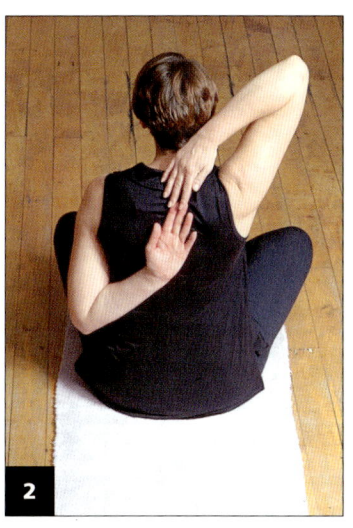

Arms

1. Raise your right arm above your head and drop your hand behind your back. With your left hand, gently push your elbow back until you feel a slight tension. Repeat with your left arm.

2. Now reach one arm behind your head and the other behind your back and try to clasp your hands together. Don't worry if they don't meet – some people are more flexible than others. Stretch gently for 15 seconds.

WEEK 11

You should take extra care now when doing any physical activity, including household chores, and avoid violent twisting or jerking movements. During pregnancy, the body produces a hormone called relaxin that softens the pelvic ligaments to make childbirth easier. This hormone also slackens other ligaments, leaving you vulnerable to sprains and other injuries.

What's happening to you
- If you have been suffering from morning sickness, you may now find that it is less of a problem. This is because your body is starting to adjust to the high levels of hormones circulating in your bloodstream.
- There is now more blood in your body, and this will continue to increase until about the 30th week (your blood volume will go up by 30 per cent overall). Your heart becomes stronger and more efficient at coping with its increased workload, but you will still feel breathless in the later stages as your circulatory system faces greater demands from your growing baby.

What's happening to your baby
- Although your baby's sex was decided at conception, it is only now that the external genitals are starting to develop.
- As the baby's neck muscles and bones develop, the head, which is still large in relation to the rest of his body (about one third the size) will start to lift off the chest.
- By the end of the 11th week, the rest of the baby's organs are fully formed inside the torso – during the rest of the pregnancy they simply grow bigger – so your baby is now virtually safe

Baby at 11 weeks

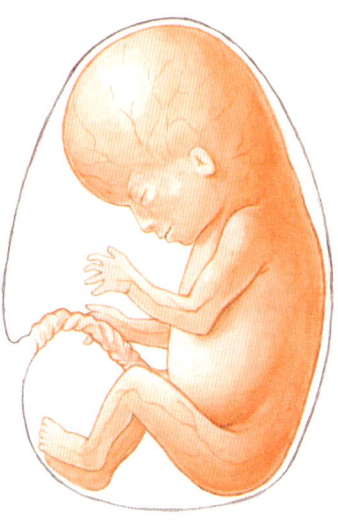

from any risk of congenital abnormalities.
- Although your baby moves around quite vigorously at times, he or she is still too small for these jerky actions to be felt by you.
- Your baby is now exercising the muscles that will eventually be used for breathing and swallowing.
- Your baby swallows amniotic fluid and excretes this as urine.
- Your baby practises the sucking reflex ready for breastfeeding – the lips come together, the forehead wrinkles and the head turns, searching for an imaginary nipple.

FACT BOX
When exercising, don't let your pulse exceed 120 beats per minute (bpm). If it does, rest until your pulse drops to below 90 bpm.

Turn the page for stage 2 of these exercises

EXERCISE – PART 2

IT IS BETTER for you and your baby to do light, daily exercises than to reserve longer and more strenuous sessions for the weekend. Just ten minutes a day can pay dividends. The simple exercises shown on these pages improve muscle tone and should only be done after completing the limbering up routine on the previous pages.

These exercises, which are based on yoga positions, have been shown to be gentle but effective. Janet Balaskas, who runs the Active Birth Centre in London, has been recommending them to pregnant women for many years with great success.

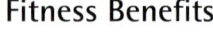

Fitness Benefits

Although exercise may be the last thing you feel like doing, there are many advantages to starting a gentle fitness routine now. Why should you exercise?

• Pregnancy symptoms (cramp, backache, constipation and sleeplessness) may be alleviated.

• You will meet other like-minded mums at prenatal exercise classes.

• A feeling of well-being follows any exercise, due to the release of natural mood-enhancing chemicals called endorphins.

• Labour will be easier, and can be quicker (see also pelvic floor exercises on pages 54 and 55) and you will be less fatigued during labour.

• You will return to your prenatal shape more quickly and easily after the birth.

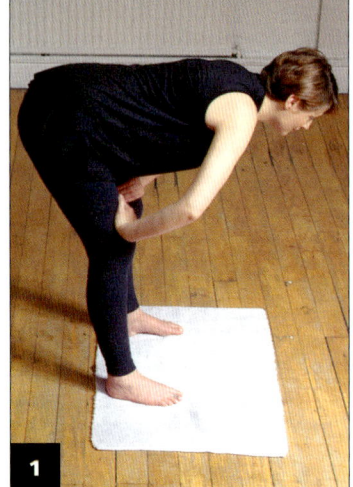

SAFE EXERCISING – You're not in a marathon!

Aerobic exercise has the most beneficial effects on health. This is any moderate level of exercise – sustained for 20 minutes or more – that raises the heart and breathing rate a little. Choose gentle forms of aerobic exercise such as walking, swimming or using a static exercise bicycle.

• **WALKING:** Regular walks of a mile or more are great for circulation and digestion. Wear wide, comfortable, flat shoes and try not to slouch. You may find walking difficult in the late stages of pregnancy.

• **SWIMMING:** Ideal for pregnant women as you exercise every muscle in your body while the water takes the weight off your back and legs. Don't feel you have to race or swim lengths.

• **YOGA:** A gentle form of exercise that is ideal for pregnancy, and one you can safely take up even if you have never done it before – the exercises on these pages are based on simple yoga positions.

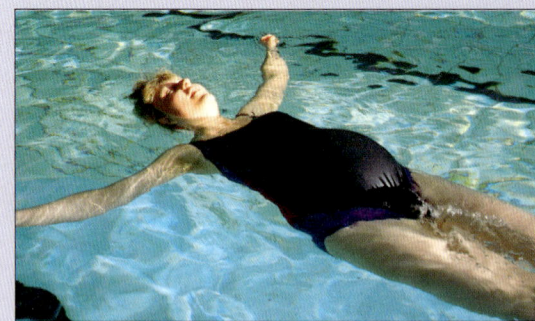

AVOID THESE ACTIVITIES

Some activities should not be attempted in pregnancy, especially during the later stages.

• **HIGH-IMPACT:** Avoid activities such as jogging and step aerobics that place a lot of strain on the back and joints.

• **WEIGHT-TRAINING:** Avoid carrying heavy weights – including backpacks – as this can cause muscle and ligament damage, raise blood pressure, and place excess strain on the abdomen.

• **HIGH-RISK:** Activities such as skiing, horse riding and contact sports are inadvisable as your weight distribution is changing and the risk of falls is much greater. Any fall on your abdomen may harm you and your baby.

• **SIT-UPS:** Avoid exercises that put pressure on your uterus or strain your abdominal muscles. In the later stages of pregnancy, when getting out of bed can be difficult, roll on to your side and use your arms to help you (see pages 68 and 69).

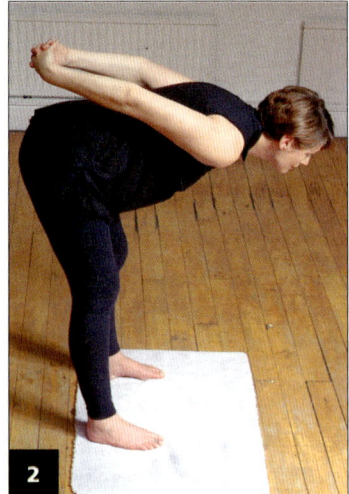

Forward bend

1. Hold your arms behind your back, with your feet shoulder-width apart. Bend forwards slowly from the hips, and breathe deeply a few times, then rise.

2. If it feels comfortable, you can raise your hands while you are bending down. Don't try to stretch too far.

Back twist

1. Lie on your back. Keeping your shoulders flat on the floor and your right leg straight, raise your left knee and swing it over to the right. Now swing it back to the middle for a short rest.
2. Repeat with your right knee. Repeat ten times.

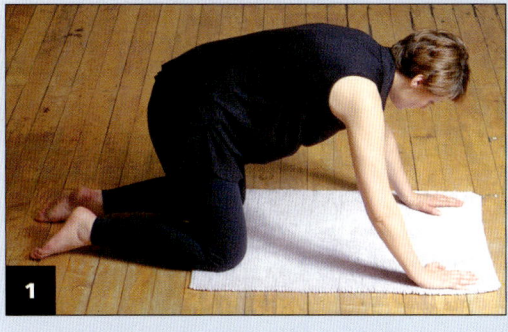
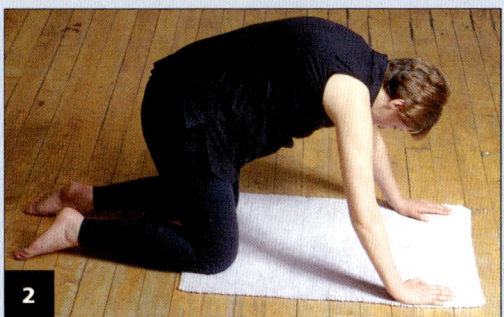

Tummy tuck

1. Kneel on all fours, with your knees shoulder-width apart.
2. Clench your buttocks and tuck in your pelvis. Repeat this action several times.

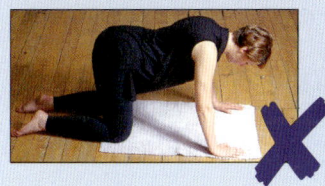

WARNING
Don't let your back sink down

Lower back stretches

1. Lie flat on your back with the soles of your feet and the palms of your hands pressing against the floor. Lift your pelvis until only your neck and shoulders are touching the floor, then lower slowly.
2. Hug both your knees together, keeping your pelvis on the floor.
3. Hug one knee, keeping the other leg straight on the floor. Now hug the other knee.

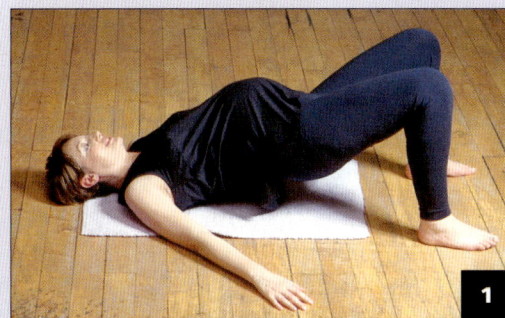
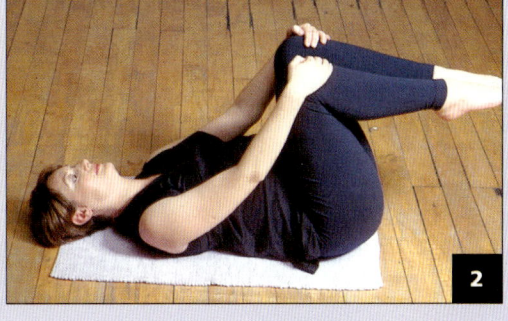
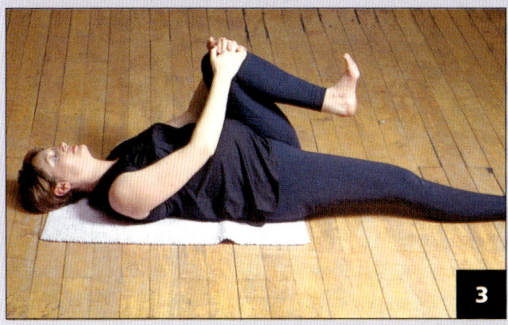

WEEK 12

Antenatal classes tend to get booked up early, so now is a good time to call in at your hospital and find out what is available in your area.

What's happening to you

• You may now notice that your weight and abdominal shape is changing, but others probably won't be aware just yet.

• Your uterus, which is getting bigger all the time, can now be felt above your pubic bone.

What's happening to your baby

• Your baby responds to external stimuli, such as noise or movement, and has fully-formed eyelids, which are closed.

• As well as swallowing and breathing, your baby may have the occasional fit of hiccups! (although you won't be able to feel anything.)

• Your baby has 32 buds in his mouth from which the primary (milk) and permanent teeth will eventually form.

• The baby's heart beats between 120 and 160 times per minute, which can be heard through a listening trumpet, a doctor's stethoscope or the listening devices parents can buy.

• Your baby is now starting to produce blood cells in the bone marrow, liver and spleen, just as you do.

• The umbilical cord is now divided into three parts: one carries oxygenated blood and nutrients to your baby, the other two remove de-oxygenated blood and waste products.

FACT BOX
Exercise produces a rush of 'feel good' chemicals called endorphins that cross the placenta and have a calming effect on your baby.

Antenatal Care

NOW THAT YOU have reached the end of the first three months of pregnancy, it is time for you to see a midwife or obstetrician. These visits are important to ensure that there are no problems with your pregnancy and to give you the opportunity to ask any questions that may have been worrying you.

Antenatal care starts at this point and continues until you have had your baby. It is impossible to say whether you will see a doctor or midwife first, as procedures differ from one area to another, but quality of care should be the same wherever you are. In some areas, you will see a midwife at your doctor's surgery, while in others you may be asked to visit an obstetrician who will see you at your local hospital.

Booking in

The first visit (at 12–13 weeks) is the 'booking in' appointment. You are registered on the antenatal care system, your notes are started and a series of check-ups are arranged. Each time you go for a check-up, you will be weighed, your blood pressure will be checked, you will be asked to provide a urine sample, and there may be a brief examination of your abdomen to see how your baby is coming along. At certain intervals you will also have blood tests.

The midwife or doctor will happily address any problems or queries you may have. Midwives are qualified to deal with most problems that may occur, and can always refer to a doctor if they need a second opinion.

Notes and queries

You will be handed your medical records (sometimes called a 'co-op card') to keep

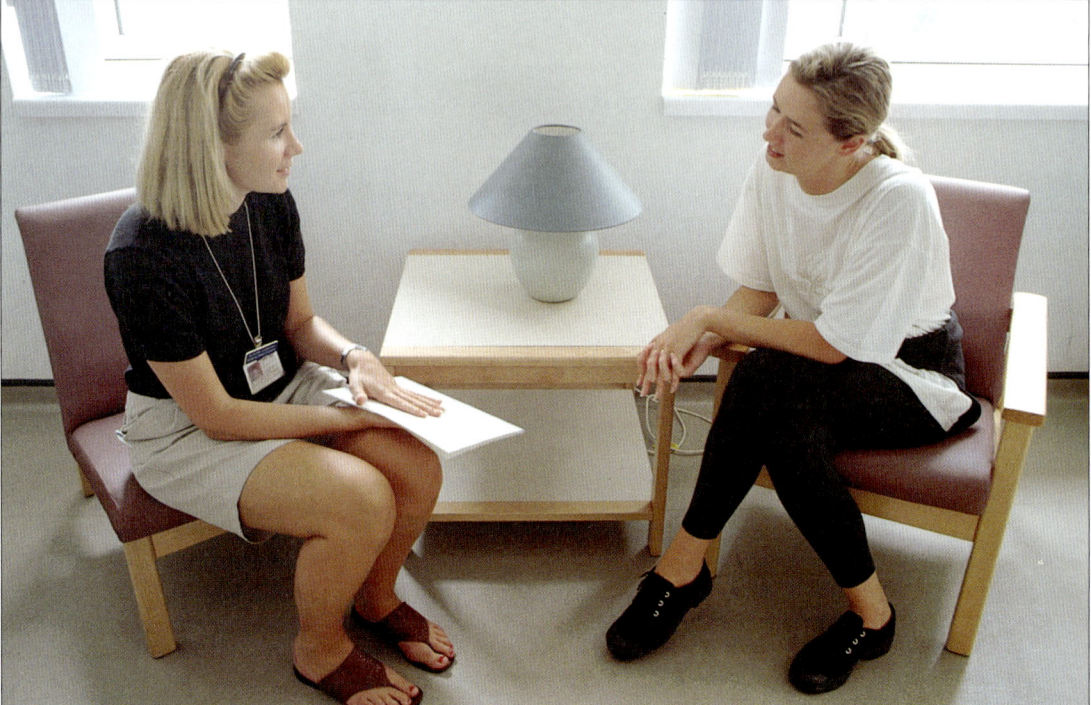

safely. These describe how your pregnancy is progressing, and contain your measurements and the results of any tests carried out. The notes are written in medical terms and can be difficult to understand. Some of the terms may even seem alarming, but in reality do not usually indicate that anything is wrong with your baby. Your midwife will be happy to explain anything on your notes you do not understand.

You should keep these notes safely and bring them along to each appointment – they will be particularly important if another doctor or midwife becomes involved in your antenatal care.

What the tests are for

By the end of your pregnancy, you may be heartily sick of people poking and prodding you and asking you for samples of blood and urine. But it is important to bear in mind that all these checks help your doctor and midwife provide the best possible care.

Blood Sample

This gives your doctor a lot of information about your state of health. It is particularly useful for monitoring your iron levels, which can fall during pregnancy due to the extra demands being placed on your system. If this happens, you may be prescribed iron tablets, but prevention is

Your midwife keeps a record of your general health during your pregnancy.

better than cure, so you should aim to maintain a balanced diet (see pages 20 and 23).

Urine sample

This is checked for signs of diabetes. A mild form of diabetes can sometimes develop during pregnancy only to disappear again once the baby is born. Urine is also tested for protein, which can be an early indicator of pre-eclampsia. If left unchecked, this can be a serious condition that may cause problems for both mother and baby during the pregnancy.

Blood pressure

This is monitored throughout your pregnancy. As well as indicating general health, blood pressure readings can also give an early warning of pre-eclampsia. The test produces two figures. The higher one,

systolic, indicates the pressure as your heart beats. The lower one, diastolic, shows the pressure as the heart relaxes. Moderately high blood pressure, or hypertension, is over 140/90. Pregnant women generally have a low blood pressure.

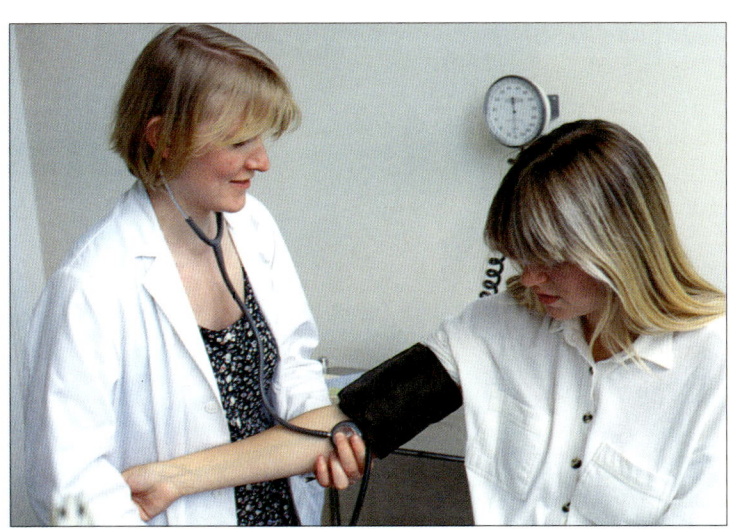

Blood pressure monitoring provides an important health check and should be carried out throughout pregnancy. An average reading for a pregnant women is 120/70.

CASE NOTES

My first antenatal visit

Jennifer is 28 and she is 3 months pregnant with her first baby:

'I was a bit nervous at first because they had to take a blood sample, and it always takes ages to find a vein. I had an easy time during the first few months, and I didn't suffer from morning sickness or anything so I didn't have any special questions to ask. The midwife let me listen to the baby's heartbeat through a special monitor, which was a real thrill.

My husband was too busy at work to come for the first visit, which was a shame as he should have been there to also hear the heart. I walked home in a bit of a daze – listening to my baby really brought home the fact that I was really going to have a baby.'

WEEK 13

You are now starting to catch up with your body's increased workload and will be feeling more energetic as your body gets more used to being pregnant.

What's happening to you

• Around this time, or sometimes a little later, a dark line, known as the linea nigra, starts to appear down the middle of your abdomen. It gets darker and more pronounced until after the birth, when it begins to disappear.
• Your nipples and areolae are becoming even darker as your breasts continue to prepare for feeding your baby.
• Your uterus is now the size of a grapefruit and can be felt above the pelvic bone.

Mother and uterus at 13 weeks

What's happening to your baby

• The fetus is really starting to look like a baby now as the arms and legs develop and are more in normal proportion with the head and body.
• Your baby's body has grown fine, downy hair, called lanugo.

• Important connections are being made between the baby's brain, muscles and nervous system – in fact, by this time your baby has as many nerve endings as you do!
• By the 13th week, your baby's hands and feet are fully formed.

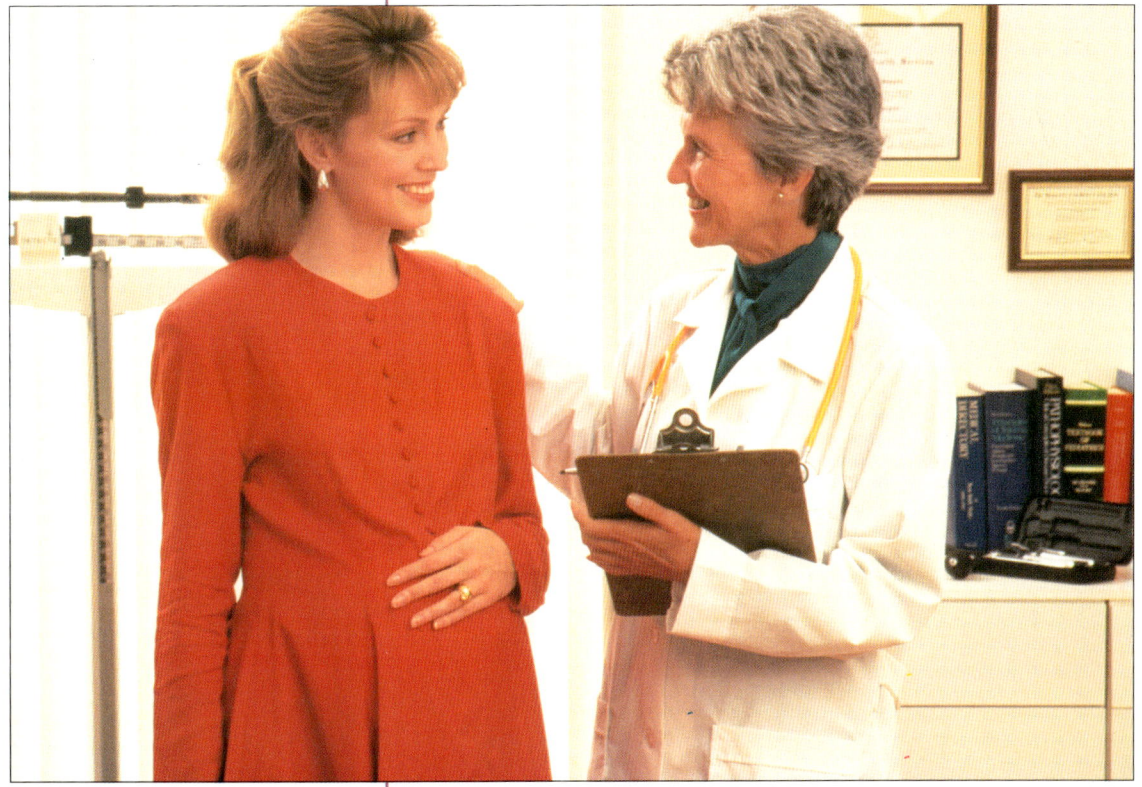

THE BIRTH SPECIALIST

THE MIDWIFE plays a key role in your antenatal care and the delivery of your child. She is also your primary link to all the health services caring for you and your baby. You will be able to get the most out of the services your midwife provides if you understand her role during your pregnancy and beyond.

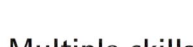

It is likely that you will have more contact with your midwife than with any other health professional in the course of your pregnancy, labour and postnatal care. Midwives are fully trained in obstetric care, delivery and postnatal recovery, and they also have the full weight of their local hospital's resources behind them. Increasingly, midwives deliver babies without the need for a doctor's intervention. If you decide you would like to have your baby at home, your midwife will organise this and will be on hand to look after you during your labour and recovery after the birth.

Continuous care

Ideally, you should be able to see the same midwife for every check-up, and then have her on hand to deliver your baby. This is not always possible, however, as your antenatal midwife may not be on duty when your baby is born.

Many health regions are now adopting the 'Domino' Scheme (DOMiciliary IN and Out) which is designed to ensure continuity of care. A Domino midwife conducts antenatal check-ups, takes the mother-to-be to hospital at the onset of labour, where she will stay on hand until the baby is born, and then takes her home again.

Multiple skills

Your midwife's primary concern is to ensure that your pregnancy and birth proceed as normally as possible – she is not just concerned when things go wrong. Don't be afraid to ask your midwife about anything connected with your pregnancy: she has the expertise to help and advise you at every stage. If you get to know your midwife and build up a relationship with her, you may feel more comfortable and relaxed in her presence, and more willing to ask her about anything that is troubling you.

After the birth, your midwife will check on your condition, to ensure there are no problems such as pain or infection from any stitches you might have had. She will also check that your baby is developing normally and give advice on practical matters such as feeding and bathing your new baby.

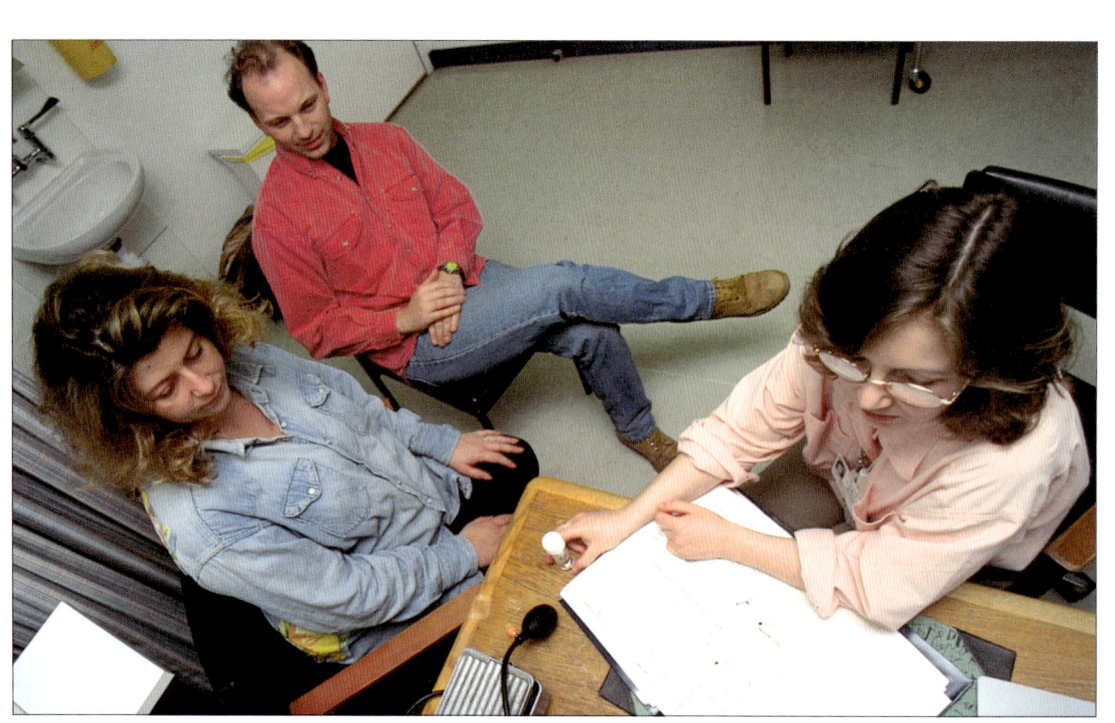

Your midwife is your professional 'birth partner', there to look after you every step of the way.

Internal and external examinations

1. Your midwife or doctor will gently place two fingers inside your vagina and feel for the neck of the womb (cervix).

2. He or she will feel internally to determine the width of your pelvis.

3. The size of your pelvis is measured by comparing his or her hand width with your pelvic opening.

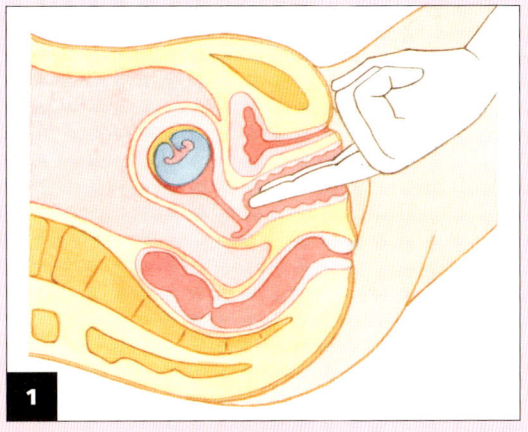

1

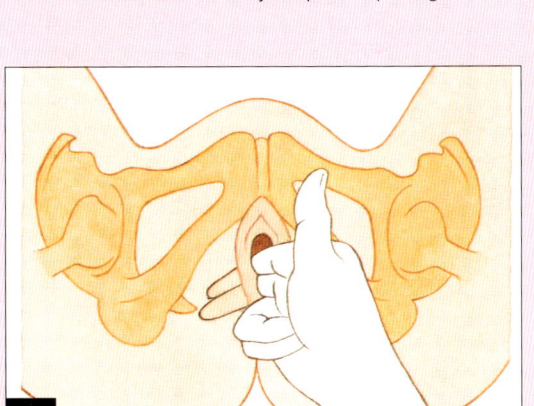

2

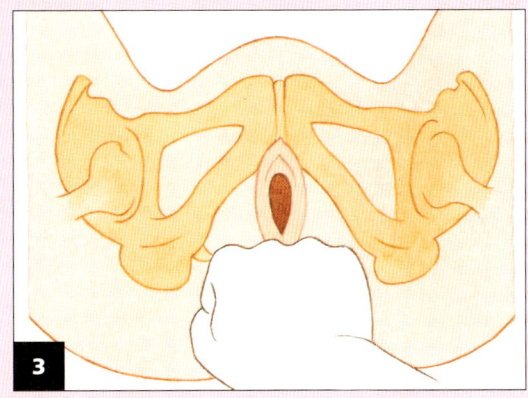

3

Your midwife will now co-ordinate all your antenatal check-ups. They will be held once a month until the 32nd week, when they will be held every fortnight. In the final month and run up to birth, your midwife will see you once a week.

What's happening to you
• You will now start to notice that all your clothes are getting much tighter around the abdomen as you fill out.
• Your uterus is now the size of a grapefruit, and is starting to show above your pelvis.

What's happening to your baby
• Inside the ball of your uterus is a baby measuring 9cm (3½in) long and really looking like a little baby.
• Hair has started to grow on your baby's head, and the eyebrows have formed.
• Sexual differentiation is beginning as the external genitalia start to develop.

Many midwives are also expanding their skills to include complementary areas of medicine. It is a good idea to check if your midwife has received any formal training in massage, aromatherapy, or reflexology as you might find these disciplines helpful, particularly in easing pain and reducing stress.

Internal and external examinations

During your regular antenatal visits you will be given physical examinations. They may be internal or external, or sometimes both.

INTERNAL: At your first antenatal visit, you will probably be given an internal examination. This is to determine how advanced your pregnancy is and how well you are equipped to deliver your

baby vaginally. This is done by checking the state of your cervix (which softens as your pregnancy progresses) and by measuring the size of your pelvis.

You will be asked to lie down and raise your knees, then your midwife or doctor will gently insert two fingers into your vagina and press on to your abdomen with the other hand. Try to relax your vaginal muscles and breathe out, as this will make the examination quicker and easier.

You may have another internal examination in the last weeks of pregnancy to determine the relative size between your pelvis and your baby's head – it should not be uncomfortable, and will in no way harm your baby.

EXTERNAL: At every visit, your midwife will gently feel your abdomen to determine the

size of your baby. These estimates are used to chart your baby's progress inside your uterus. She is feeling for the fundus, or top of your uterus, which can now be detected above your pelvic bone. At later visits, she will be feeling for the baby's head and bottom, to see how the baby is lying and to estimate the baby's weight.

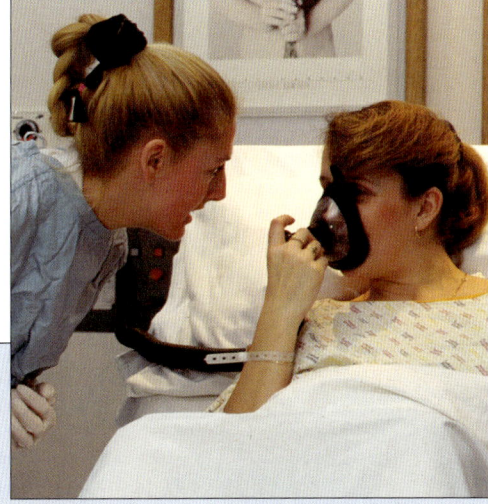

Private midwives – personal service
Although not cheap, private midwives provide a very personalised level of service, including guaranteed continuity of care and home visits for antenatal check-ups. They have all the usual facilities behind them, and can arrange for tests, liaise with your doctor or consult an obstetrician.

CLOTHING – PART 1

APART FROM the obvious change to your waistline, which is now starting to be noticeable, there are other physical changes during pregnancy that will affect what you can wear from now on. Fortunately, compared with past generations, there is now a much wider range of comfortable and attractive clothing available for mums-to-be.

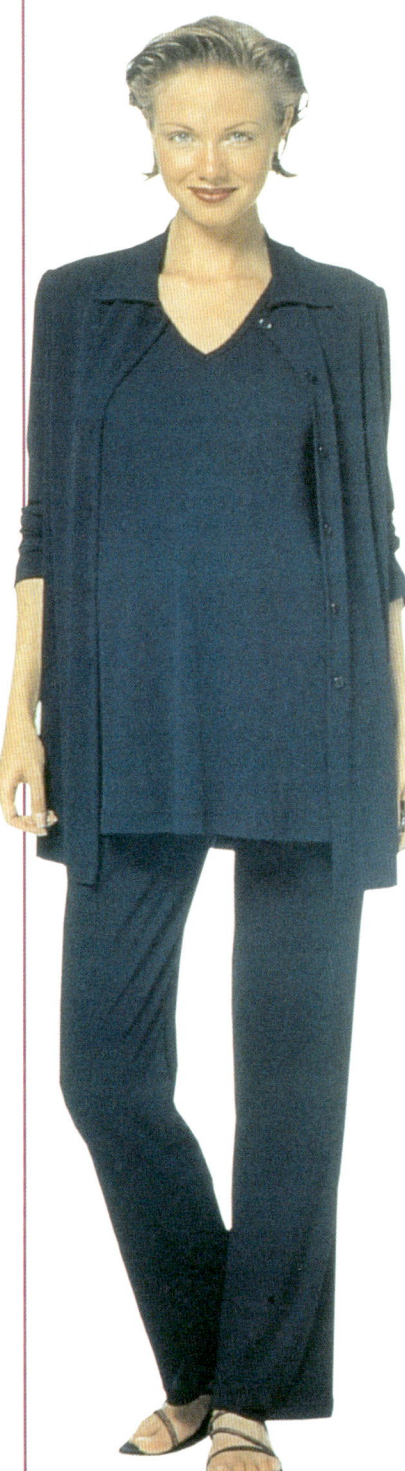

Just because your waistline is expanding and you may not be able to tie your own shoelaces in a few months' time, this does not mean you'll have to resign yourself to shapeless clothing. It is possible to pick up a few items to supplement your wardrobe and manage quite happily without breaking your bank balance. There are many more mail order companies today selling maternity wear, and you will find maternity sections in many high street clothing stores.

You will also find specialist maternity wear stores listed in your telephone directory, although these are fewer and further between. They may be more expensive but their products are good quality and the expertise of their staff can be particularly useful, especially if this is your first pregnancy.

Your changing body

When buying maternity wear it is important to know what to prepare for. Until now you may have taken for granted that your clothes will fit and feel right. But the physical changes of pregnancy can creep up on you slowly until you suddenly realise how much it matters just to be comfortable. It may help if you know what to expect.

You don't have to be a 'frump with a bump' – there is wide range of maternity wear available for you.

Overheating

Your increased blood volume is having several physical effects. One of these is that you will feel generally warmer than before and may get uncomfortably hot in warm weather. If you are going to be heavily pregnant during the summer months, plan ahead and buy some light cotton dresses with enough room for your 'bump', and enough loose material so that air can circulate.

Swelling

Fluid retention, or oedema, is a common problem for pregnant women, particularly affecting the ankles and feet. It can be very uncomfortable, especially at the end of the day if you've been standing for long periods of time. Some women also suffer aching varicose veins. Maternity tights made of cotton or wool, depending on the season, can alleviate both of these problems.

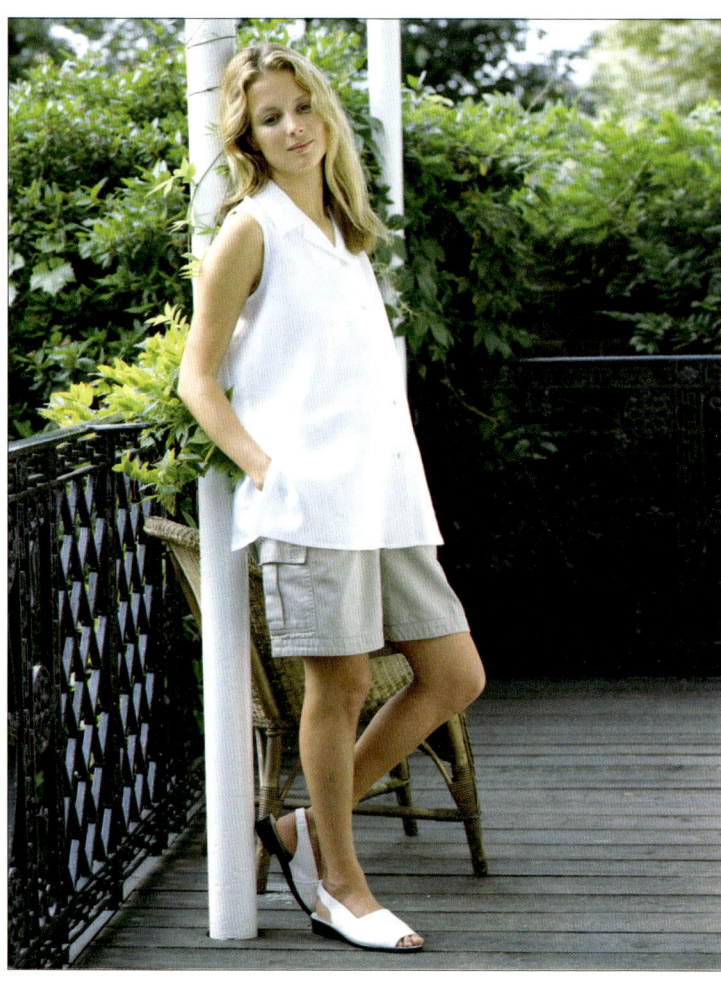

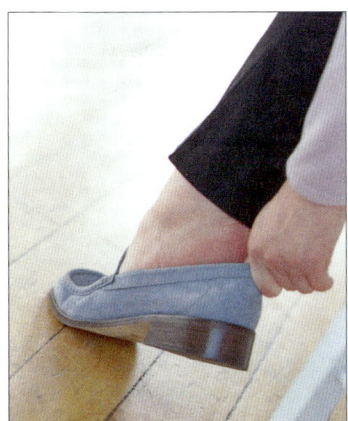

Foot problems

The increase and change in the distribution of your weight can affect your balance, so your choice of footwear is important. Avoid shoes with heels and go for flat-soled, comfortable ones that are easy to put on.

As you may not be able to tie your shoelaces during the final months of your pregnancy, consider slip-ons or shoes with Velcro fasteners. Your feet will also get noticeably wider as your pregnancy progresses, so choose wider fittings than usual.

Expansion

Your 'bump' can present the most difficult problem to clothe. Many women opt for expanders, which now come in a variety of forms from elasticated polyester waists to pleats under your ribs that you can let out as you get bigger. The advantage of such designs is that they can be comfortable throughout your pregnancy and recovery period.

For many women, a baggy T-shirt or jumper and leggings offer a cheap and effective solution. You could also try a pair of drawstring trousers, or tunics that widen at the bottom. Avoid synthetic materials as

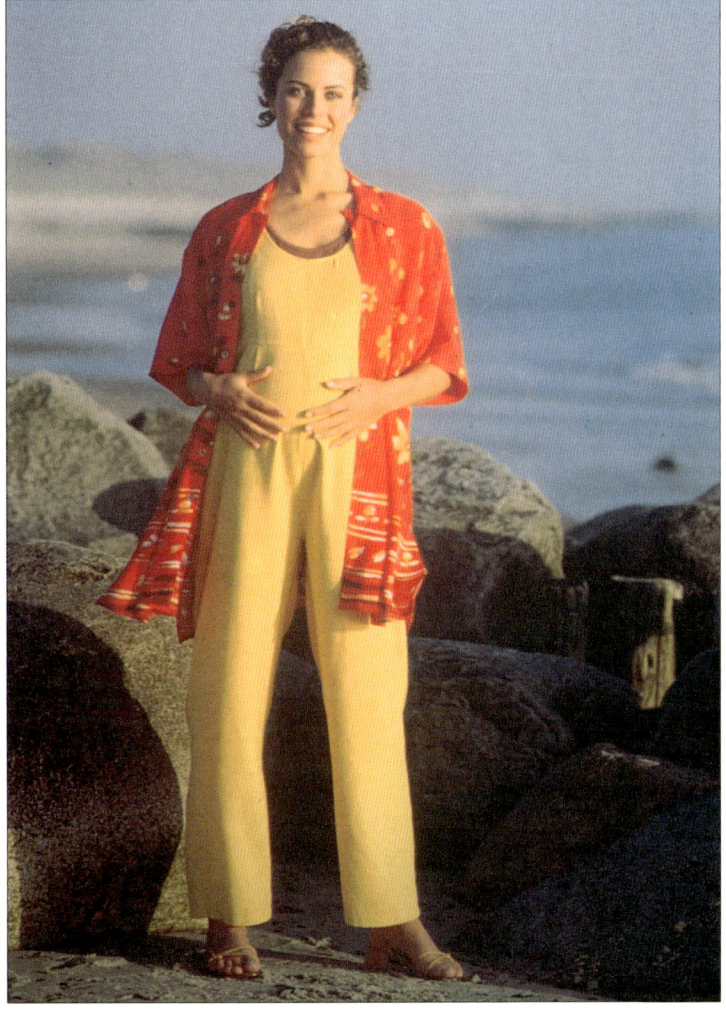

Maternity wear allows for bumps getting bigger by using expanders made with polyester or pleats.

they don't allow your skin to breathe as easily as natural fibres and can make you feel hot and uncomfortable.

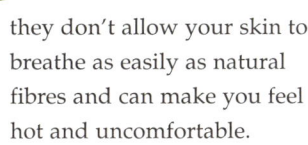

WEEK 15

Your clothes are definitely feeling tighter and it's time to start considering how to add to your wardrobe to cope with your growing 'bump'.

What's happening to you
• Your heart is now big enough to pump the extra blood (up to 30 per cent) around your body and to your placenta to keep your baby properly nourished.
• If you have freckles or moles, you may find they are turning darker.
• A small percentage of mothers develop 'chloasma', which is a dark pigmentation on the face due to high hormone levels – it used to be called 'the mask of pregnancy'. It is easily covered with makeup, and will fade after the pregnancy.

What's happening to your baby
• Your baby is now 9–10cm (3$\frac{1}{2}$–4in) – about the size of a tennis ball and weighs around 50g (1$\frac{3}{4}$ oz).
• Your baby's hair is getting thicker. Dark haired babies are now producing a dark pigment in the hair follicles.
• Your baby's skeleton is developing rapidly as the bones retain more calcium, so ensure your diet contains plenty of this mineral (see pages 20 and 21).

CLOTHING – PART 2

PREGNANCY DOESN'T mean you have to be a 'frump with a bump'. Maternity clothing has now caught up with the fashionable demands of mothers-to-be. Whether you are looking for casual clothing, formal office suits or evening wear, you can find maternity wear to suit your shape, needs and style.

You cannot escape the reality of your increasingly rapid physical changes. Your waistband will be tight about now, possibly even earlier, so it's time to think about what you can wear for the next five or six months as your pregnancy progresses further. It is important to be comfortable, especially in later months, and to give your body the kind of support and room it needs to help with the added burden of carrying a baby.

Maternity essentials

If you are on a tight budget, you may want to save as much money on maternity wear as you can. Although you may be tempted by the beautiful maternity outfits available today in high street stores or through mail order, you don't have to replace your entire wardrobe just for six months of pregnancy.

To create a practical and versatile wardrobe for your pregnancy months, make a list of the most important items you'll need. This way, you'll be able to stay comfortable and smart, without spending a fortune on new clothes that may

not be suitable after pregnancy. You may even choose to make or adapt some dresses for maternity wear, but remember to allow extra material at the front to ensure the hem is level all round.

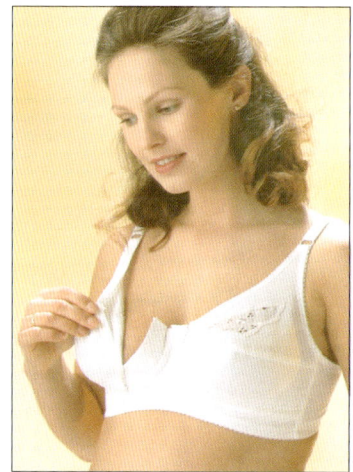

Bra

Don't try to save money on this important foundation garment (see page 26 and 27), as your breast health and your ability to regain your pre-pregnancy figure will depend on having a well-fitting maternity bra that gives you the level of support and comfort you'll need.

Maternity tights

These are specially designed with an extra section at the front to fit over your abdomen, which ensures better support and comfort.

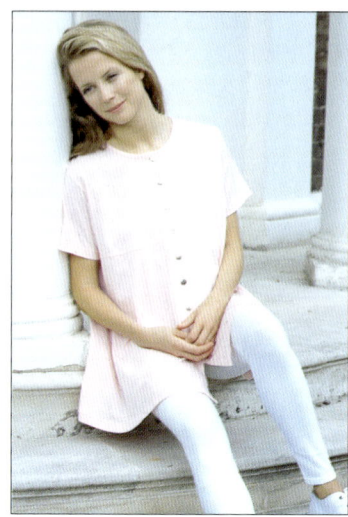

Night shirts

Even if you do not usually wear clothes in bed, you may find that a night shirt is a good investment. As your pregnancy progresses you may find it harder to get comfortable at night, in which case a soft cotton night shirt can help. Many designs also feature front openings for breastfeeding.

Leggings

Maternity types are specially designed to allow for bump expansion, either by means of a section at the front, or special panels. They also give good support to your legs – wearing leggings can help prevent or alleviate varicose veins.

Evening wear

For an occasional special night out, you can often hire formal dresses designed for pregnant women, but if you want to treat yourself, or need smart evening wear on a regular basis, there are many beautiful dresses designed with the mother-to-be in mind.

Your baby is now completely formed, and will spend the remaining time in the womb simply getting bigger. The placenta is now 1cm ($\frac{1}{2}$in) thick and roughly 8cm ($3\frac{1}{4}$in) across, and is most commonly attached to the upper part of the uterine wall.

CASE NOTES

Dressing for pregnancy

Deanna is a single mother, with her first child. She lived on a tight budget during pregnancy, and needed to find ways to save money on maternity wear.

'I borrowed big baggy T-shirts from Tim, a friend, and they were useful. I wore black cotton leggings which would stretch over my tummy until at about seven months, when they wouldn't stretch over any more. After that, I just tucked them under. It was beginning to be summer then, so I bought one light-coloured maternity smock dress that I put T-shirts on underneath. Another thing I spent money on was at the end when I got some maternity underwear, the ones that stretch over your tummy. They were just the most comfortable things ever — it was like someone holding your tummy up. Throughout the whole pregnancy I had to buy different-sized bras, but there was no way I could have avoided this. They can be expensive, but there's just no way you can live without them.'

What's happening to you
• You may now feel full of energy and vitality.
• Your skin may feel softer and more supple than usual.
• Your waistline has finally gone, and you will notice a slight rounding of your lower abdomen. This is your uterus pushing against your stomach wall as it expands to make room for your baby.

What's happening to your baby
• Your baby is about 16cm ($6\frac{1}{2}$in) long and weighs 135g (5oz).
• Your baby's skin is semi-transparent, so you would be able to see blood vessels lying just under the surface.
• Your baby has tastebuds, and the inner ears have formed – so he or she can hear everything you say.
• The legs are now longer than the arms and the fingernails and toenails have formed.
• Your baby's lungs breathe in amniotic fluid as a natural reflex. Your baby's oxygen requirements are still being met by the blood passing through the umbilical cord.

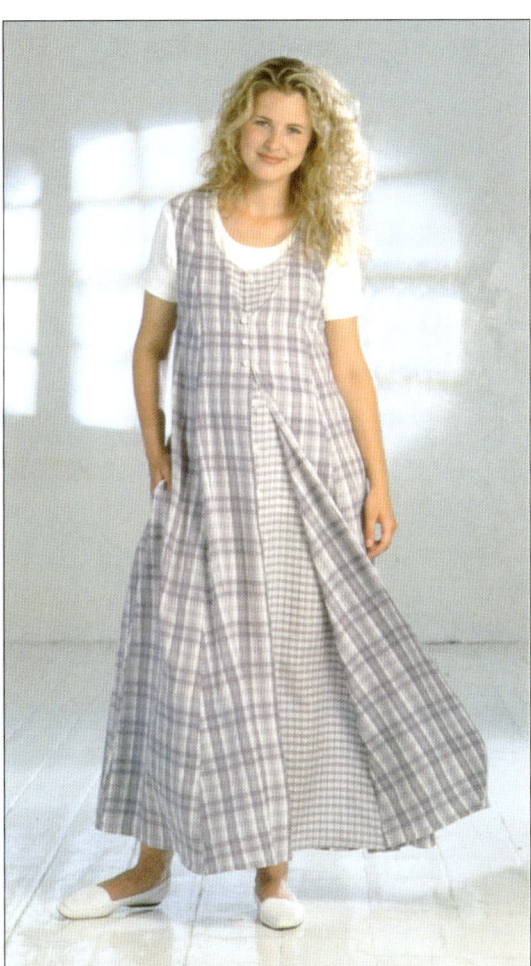

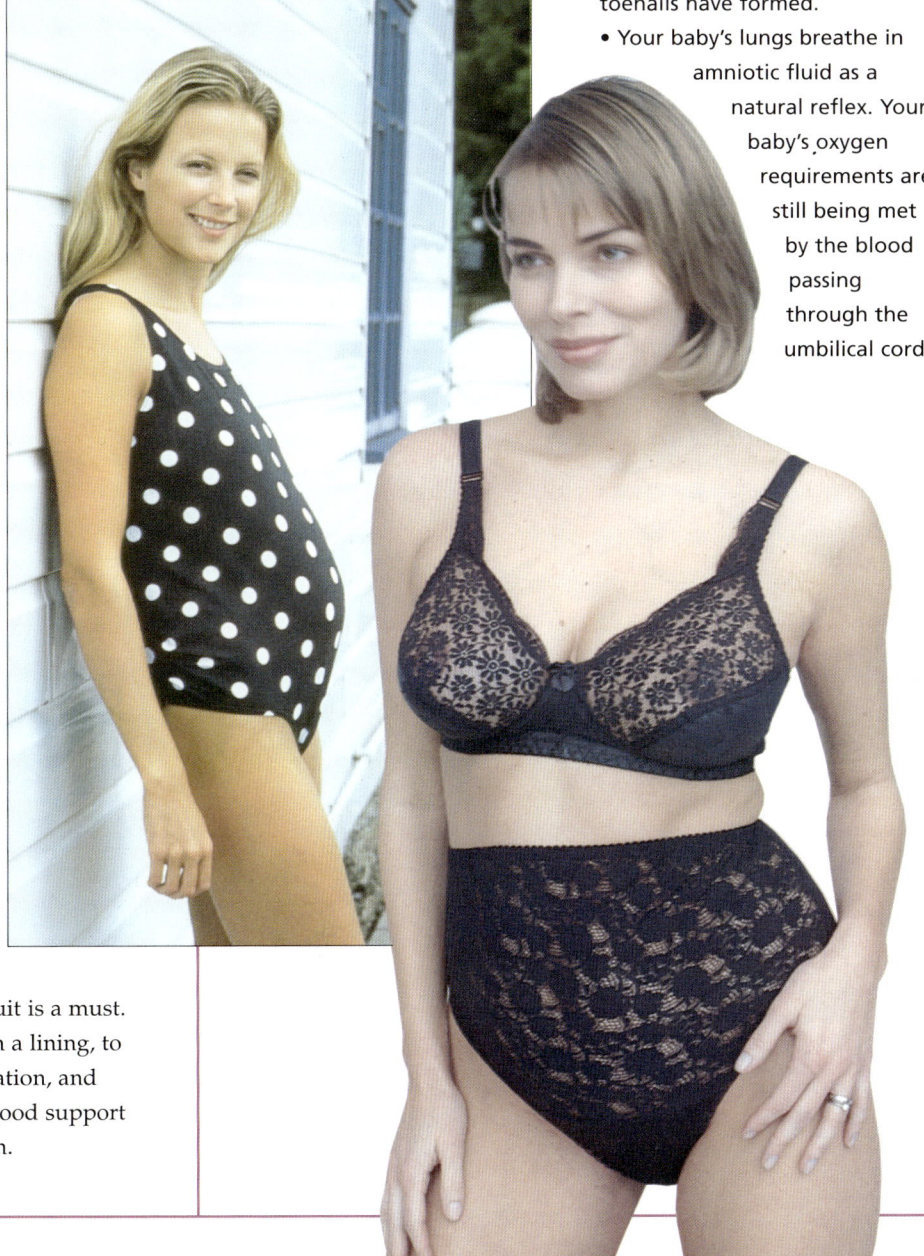

Swimsuit

Swimming provides excellent exercise during pregnancy – 'aquanatal' classes are becoming especially popular – so a maternity swimsuit is a must. Look for one with a lining, to prevent skin irritation, and which provides good support for your abdomen.

BREAKING THE NEWS

NOW IS PROBABLY a good time to reveal your happy news to a wider audience. You will not be able to conceal your pregnancy for much longer and you are past the 'danger period' for miscarriages. You will become the centre of attention but should also be prepared for the fact that your news may be greeted with mixed reactions.

Once you announce that you are pregnant you may feel that you are 'on display' both at home and at work. When people discover you are pregnant they naturally want to share in your joy. But it can make you feel as though your pregnancy is a matter for public discussion. The most important, and in many ways deeply private, development in your life has now become a major topic among friends and family, so you must be prepared for lots of questions on matters you might regard as too intimate to discuss.

In the spotlight

You may also feel that your relationship with your partner is under scrutiny.

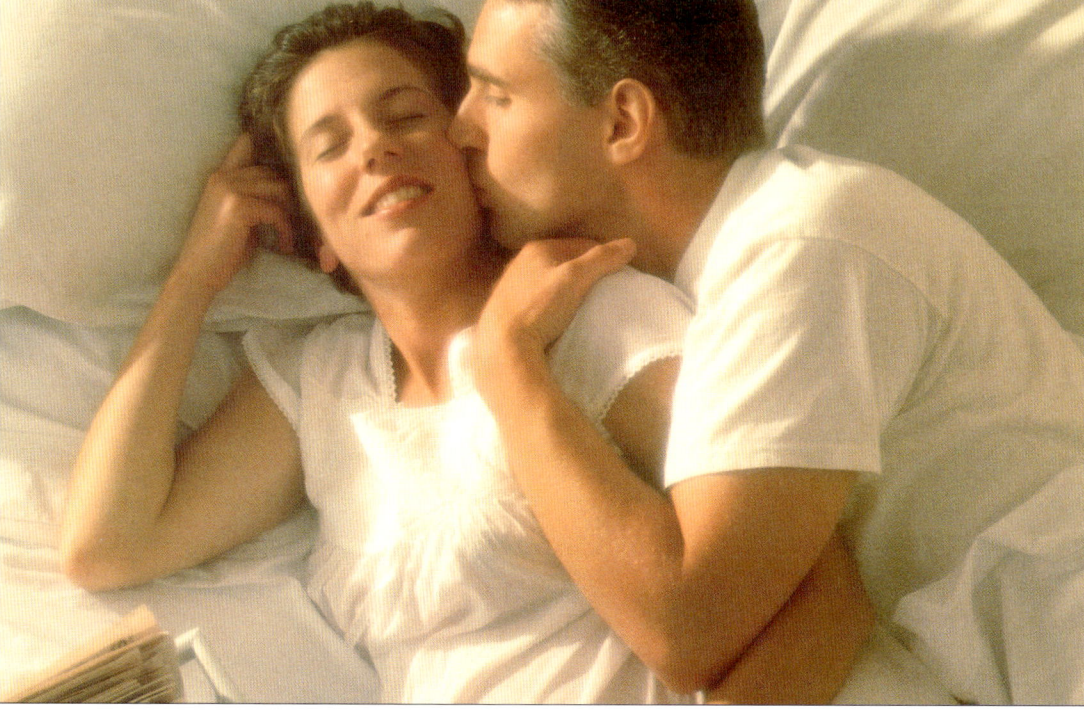

People may be wondering how he will feel about the arrival of a baby, and how you will both perform as parents. Those who are parents may want to offer advice on issues that, just at this moment, seem distant and unimportant.

Don't take all this attention to heart – if you handle it well this can be an especially joyous time for you

As the bearer of glad tidings, you can expect friends and family to be overjoyed at the news.

and your partner as the people you care about respond positively to your news. Their interest in your new family is a natural reaction, and can help you both to adjust to the idea of becoming parents.

Undercurrents

You can also expect some mixed reactions to your news, which might surprise you at first. Not everyone will feel that your pregnancy is a cause for celebration. You may even detect an undercurrent of ill feeling from one or two people, although they will be careful not to upset you. They don't feel badly towards you but, for a

Pregnancy is a magical time to share with your partner – many feel much closer during this time.

variety of reasons, are reacting to the fact that you're about to have a baby.

Your manager at work, for instance, will have to find someone to cover for you during your maternity leave, or ultimately have to replace you, if you decide not to come back to work at all. Bosses are obliged to meet the statutory maternity requirements, but may still resent it as an added burden. Others you meet at work or socially may not have been so

WEEK 17

You may now be starting to feel the baby move, which is known as 'quickening'. Second-time mothers are usually aware of fetal movement at an earlier stage, so don't worry if you haven't felt your baby move yet – you will within the next few weeks. At first, your baby's jerky movements will feel like 'butterflies', or a slight fluttering in your abdomen.

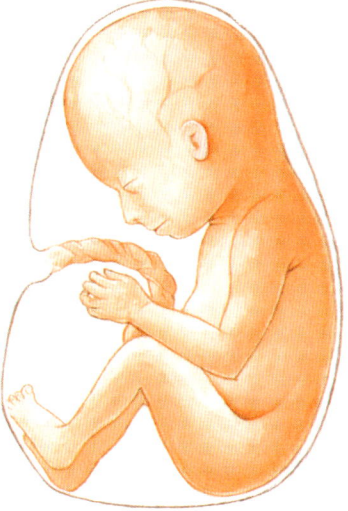

Baby at 17 weeks

What's happening to you

• You have a tendency to sweat more and may find that your nose gets blocked more often than usual.

• You may feel a slight pain or discomfort in your side when you move. This is a sign that the ligaments attached to your uterus are being stretched slightly. It is not usually a problem and will go away when you rest, but talk to your doctor or midwife if it gets more severe or is accompanied by other symptoms.

lucky with starting their own families, and this can also give rise to feelings of resentment.

Accepting motherhood

Confidence is your best ally in helping you to become the best parent you can. First-time mums often say that many of their parenting skills came quite naturally to them, especially once they started caring for their newborn. The trick is knowing that you are the best person possible to care for your baby.

Babies make good teachers – they instinctively know when something is wrong with the way you hold them, or feed him, so trust in your baby's instincts.

Health professionals are familiar with the concerns and anxieties of new mums, and will be able to give sympathetic and useful advice. Don't start worrying that you won't measure up as a mum, but simply concentrate on having a healthy pregnancy and preparing for the new family member.

FACT BOX Now that the tiny bones inside your baby's ears have formed, your baby can hear your heart, your voice, and even the blood flowing round your body.

What's happening to your baby

• Your baby's body is starting to lay down brown fat, a deposit of fatty tissue, particularly around the torso. This will help the baby regulate body temperature after the birth. One of the reasons that premature babies are so vulnerable is that they are born before they have built up sufficient deposits of brown fat to keep them warm.

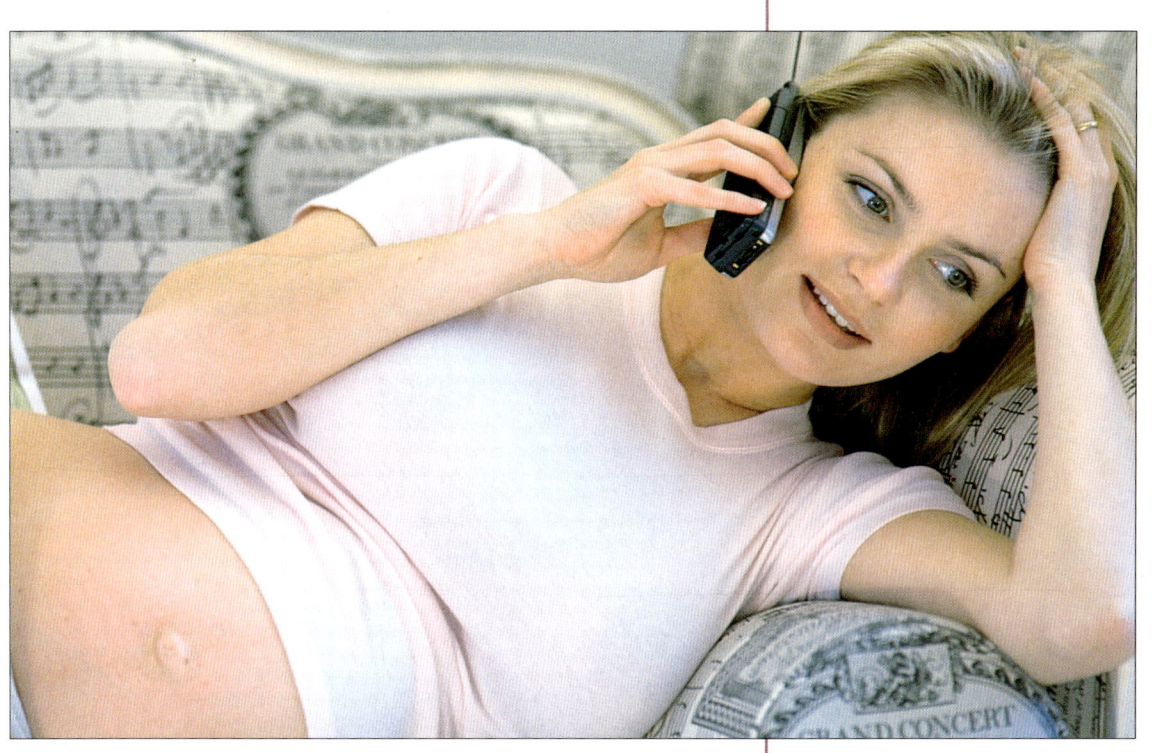

If you have friends or family members who are already parents, they will become an invaluable source of advice and reassurance to you.

FACT BOX If you believe your job puts your baby's health at risk, you have the right to ask to be moved to a safer job, provided one is available. Seek legal advice if in doubt.

YOUR FIRST SCAN

FACT BOX

By law, mothers-to-be must be allowed a reasonable amount of time off to attend medical appointments and antenatal classes. Your local Citizen's Advice Bureau can advise you on your rights.

BETWEEN 16 AND 20 weeks, you will be offered your first ultrasound scan at your local hospital. This is a thrilling and emotional time for parents as they 'see' their growing baby for the first time. The development of ultrasound has been a major breakthrough in antenatal care, so it is helpful to understand its uses.

During a normal pregnancy, you can expect to have two or three ultrasound scans over five months. Being able to 'see' inside your uterus without risk to the baby gives doctors and midwives accurate information to help them assess your pregnancy. They can examine your baby and take measurements, and also look at the placenta to check its size and position.

Safe sounds

Ultrasound is considered to be harmless for you and your baby. It works by bouncing ultrasonic sound waves off your internal organs, including your uterus and the fetus. The echoes are picked up by the scanner and converted into an image that is displayed on a screen. As it uses very high frequency sound waves, neither you nor your baby will be able to hear them. It is similar to the 'echo location' system dolphins use.

At the first scan, the ultrasound operator is looking to confirm your pregnancy (although it may be obvious to you), and to confirm your estimated date of delivery. This date is accurate to within one week with the help of ultrasound in early pregnancy. The operator measures the baby's length and the circumference of the head, in order to assess the rate of growth, and is also checking to see whether you are going to have twins.

Follow-up scan

The scan can detect abnormalities such as heart defects, intestinal and kidney malformations and spina bifida. But don't be alarmed if you are offered a follow-up scan soon after the last one. This doesn't necessarily mean your baby is at risk. It may simply be that the operator could not check every aspect of the pregnancy in

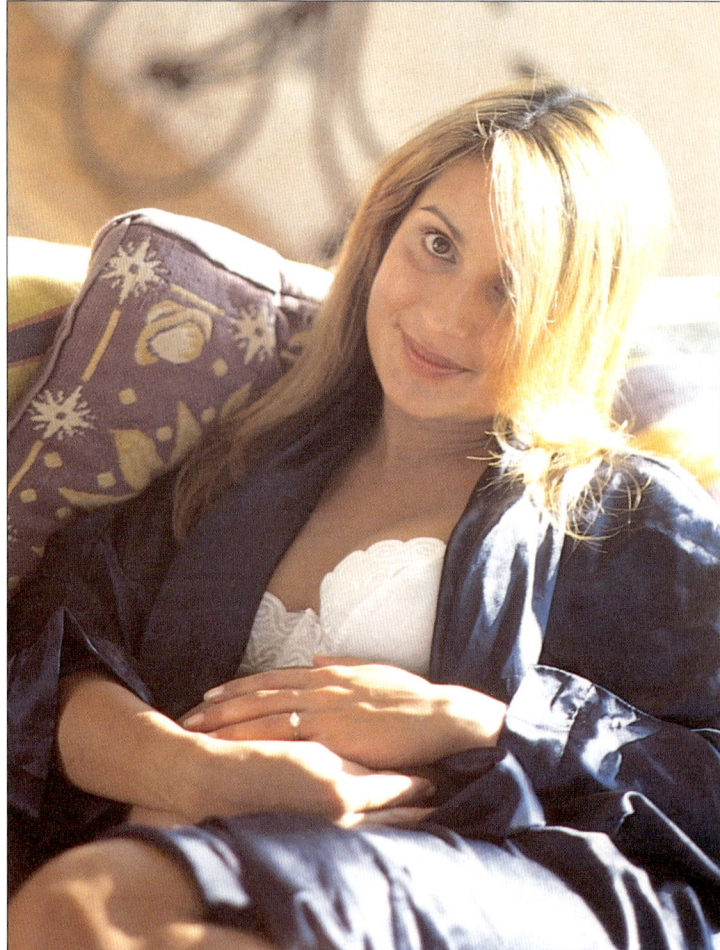

one go – important features are sometimes obscured, making it difficult to get the full picture.

If you report bleeding at any time, you may be offered a scan to check the position and condition of the placenta. Sometimes part of the placenta can become detached from the wall of the uterus (see pages 56 and 57).

Your first scan is a really exciting event, so make sure your partner comes too!

During an amniocentesis test (see pages 62 and 63), ultrasound must always be used to help guide the needle accurately so that it does not harm your baby or the placenta.

In later scans, operators compare the baby's growth rate against the average size for a baby of that age. Sometimes they may need to assess whether your baby is physically mature enough to survive outside the womb.

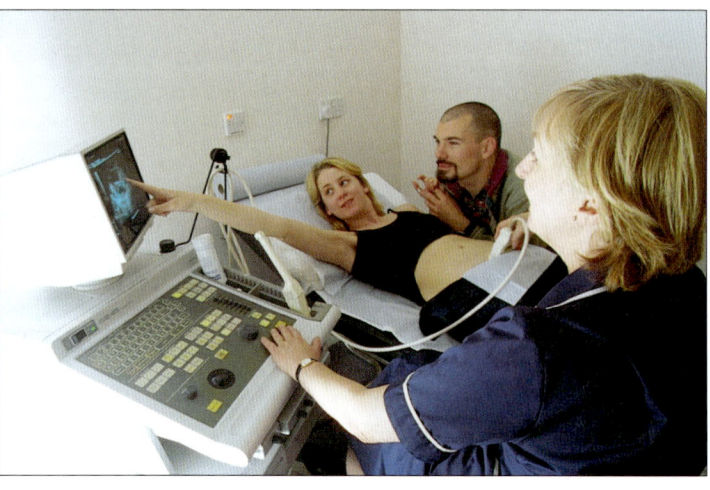

WEEK 18

The sex of your baby may now be determined by an ultrasound operator, so long as the baby's genitals are in view. If it is a boy, a penis will be visible – and the operator may be able to point it out. If it is a girl, the vaginal opening is just starting to hollow out, but this can be much harder for the operator to see.

Most hospitals will offer you a copy of the scan to take home. This is a great keepsake – your new baby's first 'picture'. Bring some money with you, as most hospitals charge a small fee for this service.

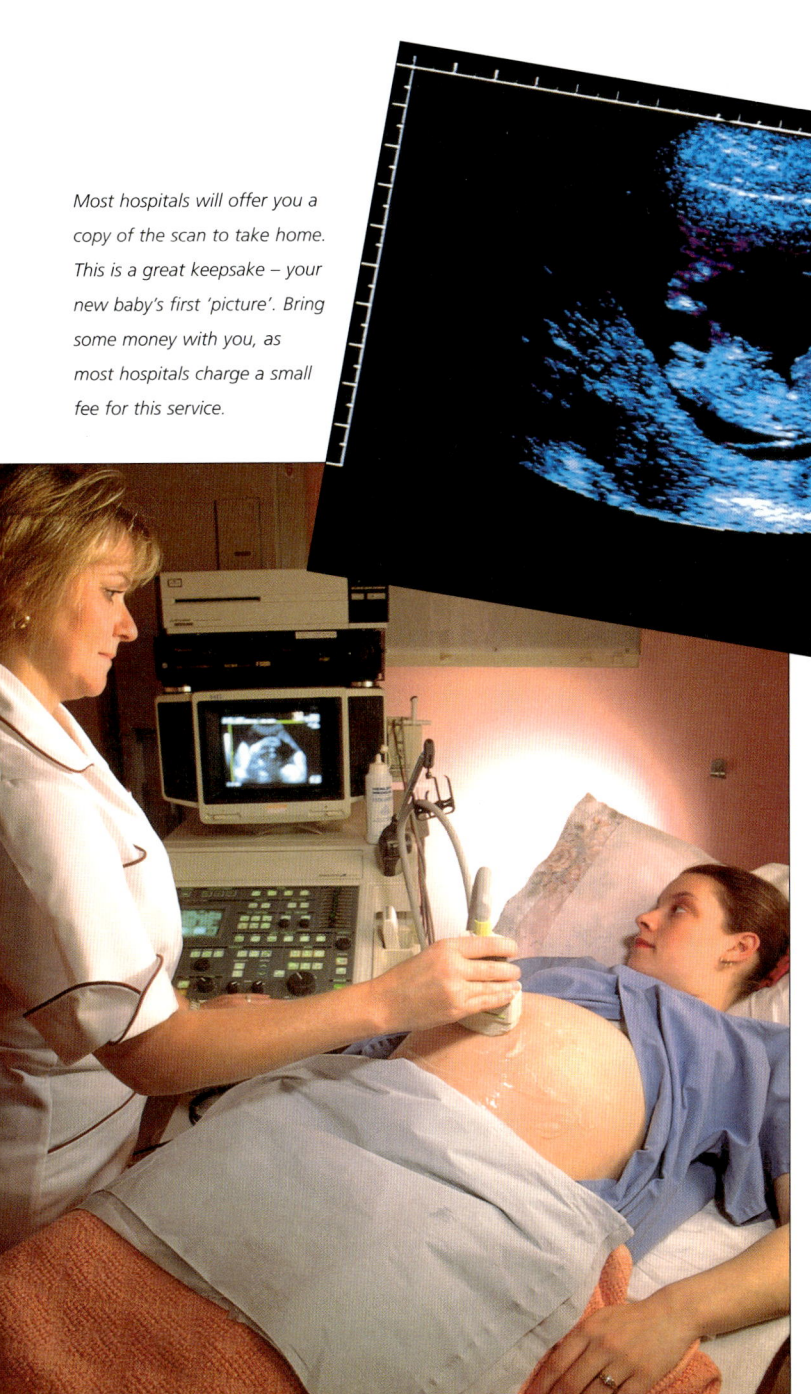

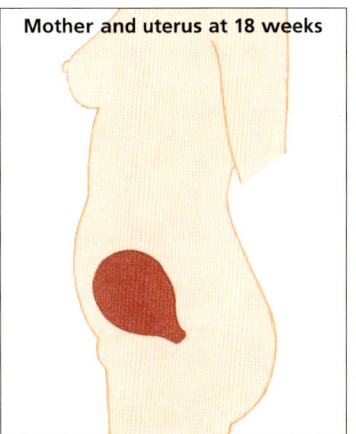

Mother and uterus at 18 weeks

What's happening to you
• You may have trouble sleeping and may need more pillows to support you so you can get comfortable.
• Your uterus is moving higher above the pelvic bone, and gradually more and more of your abdomen shows above your waistband as you develop a 'pregnant belly'.

What's happening to your baby
• Your baby may be startled by loud noises now, causing movements that you may feel.
• If your baby is a girl, she already has two ovaries with up to 7 million eggs. As she develops, she will carry fewer eggs, not more. At birth the number has dropped to about 2 million, and she will probably release around 400–500 eggs during her lifetime.

What you can expect

Before your scan, you may be asked to drink plenty of water and not go to the bathroom. A full bladder gives the scanner a clearer image, but can be an uncomfortable wait for you! You are then asked to put on a hospital gown and lie on the bed next to the scanning unit. Your abdomen is covered with gel to give better contact and stop air getting trapped between your skin and the transducer (the unit that emits the sound waves and receives their echoes).

The image is displayed on a screen and can be frozen at any time so the operator can take measurements. Don't expect to recognise your baby immediately – it can appear fuzzy and difficult to understand until the operator points out the head and limbs. After a while you will be able to identify all the baby's features.

CASE NOTES

Having a scan

Emily has been married to Mohammed for five years. They have been planning children for a long time and want a large family.

'We had been looking forward to the first scan for a while. When it was time, we were both there, but because of the position of the table to the monitor, I couldn't really have a clear view, and the picture was fuzzy and the baby was moving around a lot. My husband saw the whole thing as he held my hand, and that meant a lot to him because up to that point he hadn't really been involved – our pregnancy was just something that was going on inside me. We regretted not paying for one of the photographs when we got home, so we got one when we went for another scan. They couldn't tell us whether it was a boy or a girl because they said it was lying the wrong way round, but that suited us – we weren't going to ask anyway.'

KICK CHARTS

ALL BABIES HAVE their own unique pattern of waking, sleeping and moving inside the womb and you will soon learn to recognise yours. Midway through your pregnancy, you may be given a 'kick chart' to record your baby's movements. This will help to reassure you that your baby is healthy and all is well with the pregnancy.

By now, you will probably have felt your baby move for the first time. Second and third-time mums may have noticed this a few weeks earlier, as they may know from experience exactly what early fetal movements feel like. As your baby grows bigger and stronger, you will have no trouble identifying the kicks and prods made by him or her squirming and wriggling inside you. You will even be able to see tiny bulges in your abdomen as the baby pokes out a hand or a foot – your partner will be able to see them too.

Peak activity

Babies move between 100 and 700 times a day on average, depending on what stage the pregnancy has reached, but you will not always be able to detect these movements. This activity peaks at around week 32, then tails off as the baby becomes too large and space too restricted to have much freedom of movement. Even then, you will still be receiving sharp kicks or pokes from the baby's elbows or bottom. Sometimes you will be able to see the baby 'swim' from side to side.

Counting the kicks

A healthy baby is one that moves around inside you. This is not to say that the more a baby moves, the healthier he or she will be, but there is a minimum number of fetal movements per day that generally indicates all is well inside you. You may be given a kick chart to monitor these movements. You will be asked to mark at what time between 9am and 9pm you felt your baby's tenth movement. If you feel less than ten, you should mark exactly how many movements you did feel during that 12 hour period.

If the baby seems inactive, you may be advised to get in touch with your midwife or doctor who may ask you to come into hospital for a scan. It does not usually mean that anything is wrong, but they will just want to make sure. Ten movements is only a guideline, so you should also call your doctor or midwife if you feel that your baby's movements are unusually low – only you can really tell what is and isn't normal for your baby.

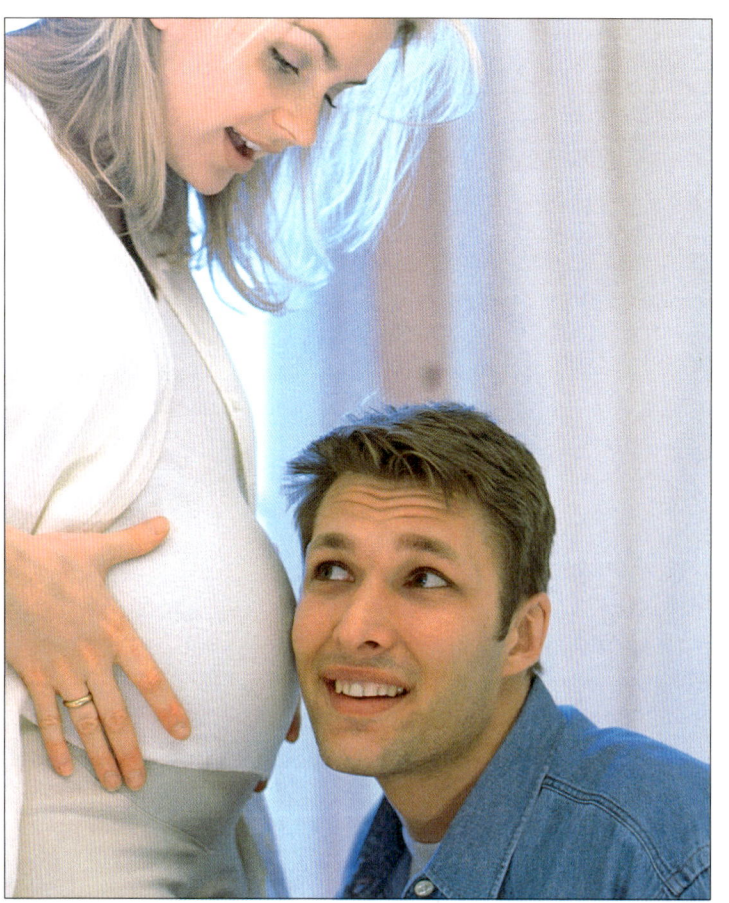

Your partner will soon be able to feel the baby move, and it is important to include him as early as possible.

In tune with baby – responding to your moods

In a way, your baby knows what you are thinking. If you become agitated or excited, your baby is also affected as adrenaline crosses the placenta and enters the fetal bloodstream. Other emotional states, such as fear, anger, stress or anxiety, can also effect your baby's moods. You may notice the baby responds by moving more frequently when you are in a particular mood.

As your pregnancy progresses you will get to know these responses. If you are feeling particularly agitated, it is a good idea to take a rest and calm down. Concentrate on letting your muscles relax, and breathe slowly, deeply and rhythmically. Practise a calming meditation technique, such as imagining yourself lying on a deserted beach, or in a restful woodland glade. You could even try humming – your baby will hear this and be comforted.

USING A KICK CHART

Instructions – please read carefully

A 'KICK COUNT' is a way by which we can see how active the baby is, and this helps us to decide if the pregnancy is going as well as we would like.

This is what you must do

Each morning, from 9.00 am, count the number of times you feel the baby kick. When you have counted TEN kicks put a tick ✔ in the box provided for each day.

Note

If you have not felt 10 kicks in a 12-hour period, it is important that you telephone the labour ward.

WEEK 19

If you haven't felt your baby move yet, you certainly will very soon. You are most likely to recognise these movements when you are sitting down or lying quietly. There is no need to worry if you don't feel a movement immediately – your baby is probably resting too.

What's happening to you
• You may notice the beginnings of stretch marks across your abdomen, just above your hips. Skin creams may help reduce these marks, and they will fade somewhat after the birth.

• Some mums also notice tiny blood vessels near the surface of their skin, particularly on their face and upper torso. These are harmless – they are known as spider naevi and will vanish once your body returns to normal after the birth.
• You may find that other parts of your body, such as your bottom, start to increase in size, and not just your breasts and abdomen.
• Increased vaginal discharge is common at this time and, if very heavy, you may need to wear sanitary pads. Don't be tempted to douche, and avoid using bath salts or foams.

What's happening to your baby
• Your baby now weighs around 0.5kg (1lb), and is 18cm (7in) long from the top of the head to the rump.
• Your baby is kicking more, and can grasp and suck. During a scan, you may notice that the baby moves so much that the image can be quite difficult to follow. You may even see him or her sucking a thumb.
• Your baby's nerve connections are developing. The baby's movements are helping to strengthen nerve signals to the muscles.

Name: _____ Expected date of delivery: _____

Hospital No: _____ Date: _____

FETAL MOVEMENT RECORDING

Starting at the same time every day, mark the square that covers the time at which you felt your baby's tenth movement.

Time	M	T	W	T	F	S	S
9am							
10am	✔		✔				
11am		✔		✔			
12md							
1pm							
2pm							
3pm							
4pm							
5pm							
6pm							
7pm							
8pm							
9pm					✔		

If you feel less than ten movements within 12 hours, up to 9pm, make a mark in a box here against the number you have felt.

	M	T	W	T	F	S	S
9							
8							
7						✔	
6							
5							
4							
3							
2							
1							
0							

FACT BOX
Allergy conditions, such as hay fever, can get worse during the second trimester. There are safe medications you can use so ask your doctor or pharmacist to recommend one.

FATHER FIGURE

THE IDEA of becoming a father may affect your partner deeply, although at first he may not be conscious of just how much. It can strengthen your relationship with your partner if you can try to understand his feelings at this time, and discover the best way to help him adjust to his new role.

This is an important time for your partner. He will probably have just felt the baby's first kick through your tummy, and have noticed how much larger you've become around your middle over the last month. It is now beginning to sink in that he'll be a dad in four months' time.

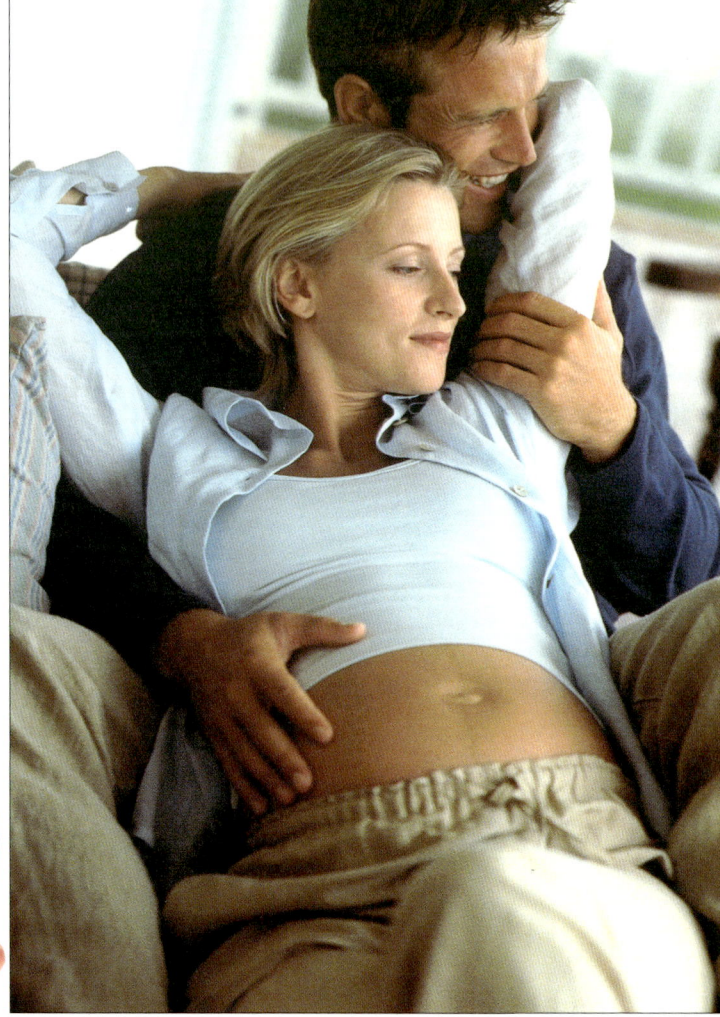

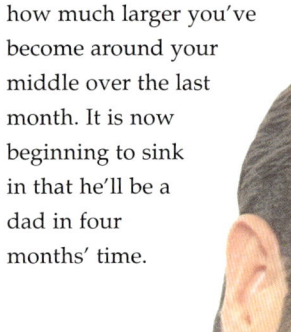

Getting involved

Until your baby is born, your partner can only really get involved through antenatal classes and by preparing for the birth. If he seems enthusiastic, encourage him to make time to join you as often as possible for your antenatal classes. Get him to take part in your breathing exercises, and to join any partner classes that your hospital may run, or may be run independently in your area.

You will need to start preparing the nursery before you are too big to move around easily, so make sure he gets involved too, and let him make some of the decisions. It has been suggested that fathers who take an active role in their partner's pregnancy from the

Being a father is often said to be the best thing that happened to a man, so don't be surprised if you suddenly make your partner the proudest man alive.

WEEK 20

Your normal bra will no longer fit you as your breasts get bigger in preparation for breastfeeding. If you have not already done so, you should now have a fitting for a maternity bra, otherwise you will feel uncomfortable and your breasts will not recover their shape as well as they should after you finish breastfeeding.

What's happening to you

Baby at 20 weeks

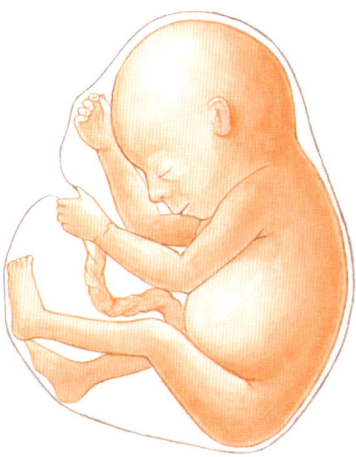

• Your gums are softer than before as a result of the pregnancy hormones. Be extra careful when brushing your teeth, and consider switching to a brush with softer bristles. You are also more prone to dental decay, so be even more meticulous about brushing and flossing after you eat. If you haven't already done so, book a dental appointment now.

• You may find that your baby is more active in the evenings, and your partner will soon be able to feel movement through your abdomen. This is a thrilling sensation for him, so don't be surprised if he wants to spend all day listening to your tummy.

What's happening to your baby

• Your baby is now 25cm (10in) long.

• Your baby is coated in a waxy substance called vernix. This protects the baby's delicate and wrinkled skin from the effects of being suspended in amniotic fluid for such a long time – imagine what your skin would look like if you took a bath for nine months.

beginning adapt more quickly and easily to the responsibilities of parenthood. They are also much more likely to be supportive and helpful during pregnancy and labour, so it is in the best interests of both you and your baby to get dad in on the act as soon as possible.

Sharing feelings

It is also important that you talk over any misgivings he may be feeling towards his impending responsibilities. If he is a first-time father, he may be suffering anxiety over his ability to support you both. He may worry that the baby will take up all your time, or that a newborn infant will rule both your lives and he won't be able to spend the amount of time with you, or with his friends that he is used to. The saying 'three's a crowd', although a cliché, does have some bearing on this matter.

Take care that once the baby arrives your partner does not feel left out as you concentrate on getting to know your newborn. Include your partner as much as possible, and let him

look after the baby some of the time so that he has a chance to bond as effectively as you already have. Perhaps you could express milk and let dad feed the baby from a bottle. Remember, he has not had the benefit of carrying the baby around for nine months, and so has had a much later start in getting to know his child.

Although it has ups and downs, parenting brings you closer together.

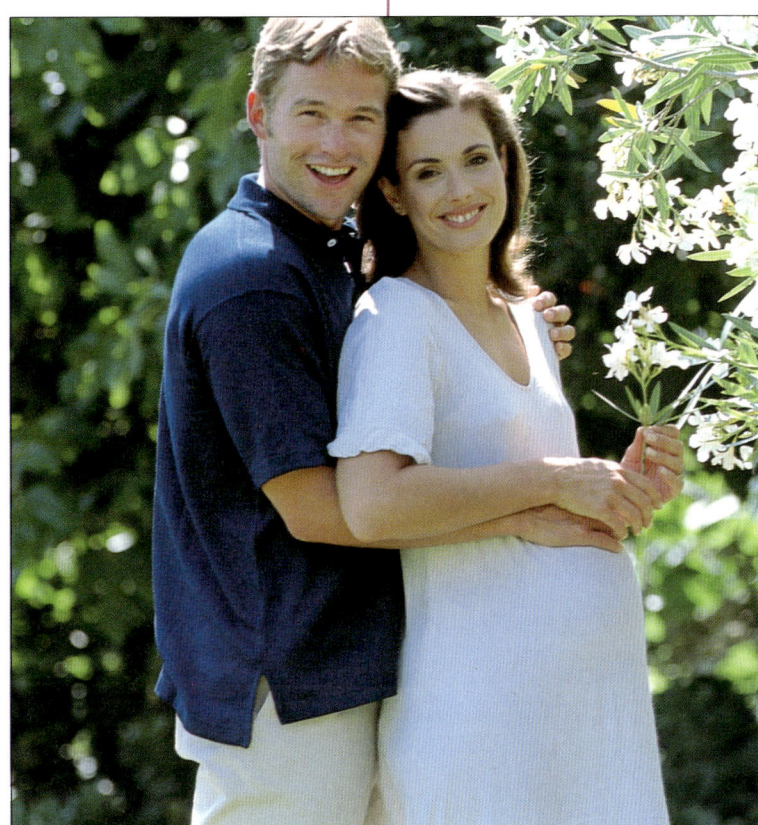

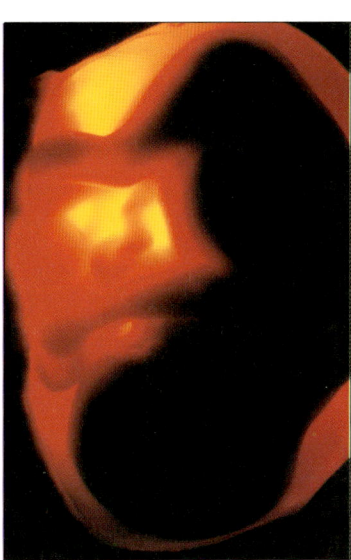

At 20 weeks, your baby will look something like the one in this picture.

HARD TO DIGEST

HEARTBURN IS a common problem for pregnant women, and can strike at any time during pregnancy. But you need not let it make your life a misery. There are simple steps you can take to reduce its frequency and severity and help you to stay as comfortable as possible over the months ahead.

Heartburn is caused by a combination of factors that are specific to pregnancy, the main one being the sheer lack of room in your insides. As your baby and uterus expand and push upwards, there is less room available for your stomach. This means that acidic gastric juices are sometimes forced out of your stomach and up into your oesophagus, or 'gullet', the tube that carries food down from your throat. The oesophagus does not have the stomach's protective lining and so becomes inflamed by the gastric juices, causing the burning sensation of heartburn.

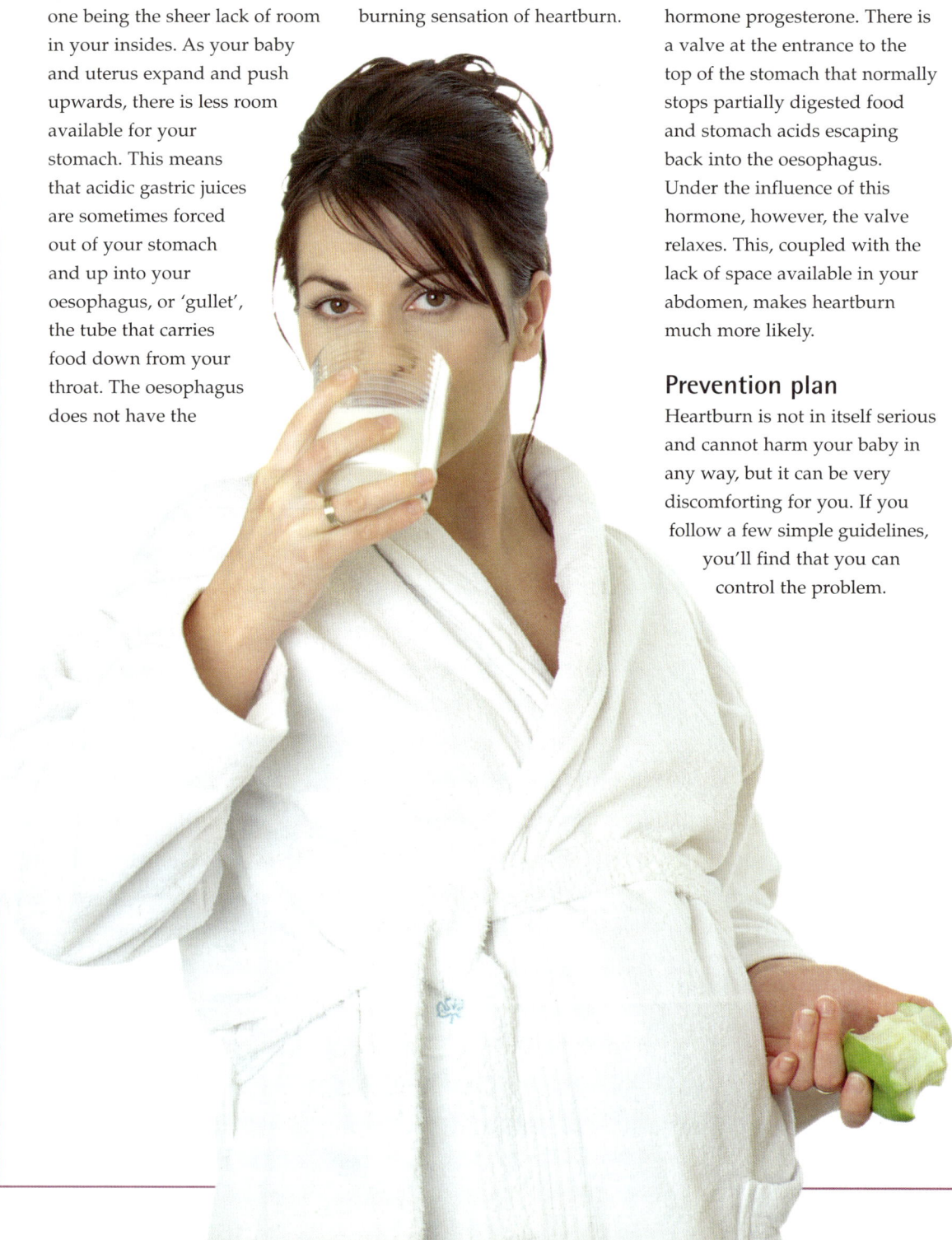

Hormonal effects

Another factor that contributes to heartburn is the effect of the hormone progesterone. There is a valve at the entrance to the top of the stomach that normally stops partially digested food and stomach acids escaping back into the oesophagus. Under the influence of this hormone, however, the valve relaxes. This, coupled with the lack of space available in your abdomen, makes heartburn much more likely.

Prevention plan

Heartburn is not in itself serious and cannot harm your baby in any way, but it can be very discomforting for you. If you follow a few simple guidelines, you'll find that you can control the problem.

Eat little and often

As your pregnancy progresses you'll find that your appetite increases in order to sustain your growing baby. This is particularly so during the last trimester as it is during the last few months that your baby puts on most weight. If you eat big meals, your stomach will be full and under greater pressure, and so much more likely to release acid into your oesophagus. To avoid this problem, try to eat smaller meals more often, even if it means dividing a meal into two portions and then finishing it later.

Drink a glass of milk

The acid in the stomach juices can be partially neutralised by the natural antacids in milk. You will find cold milk especially soothing for your oesophagus. This may be particularly effective when heartburn strikes at night.

Prop yourself up

Heartburn is more likely to occur when you are lying down to rest or sleep, particularly during the later months of your pregnancy. This is simply because the effect of gravity makes it easier for the stomach juices to escape into the oesophagus. Instead of lying all the way down when you sleep, use some pillows to prop yourself up so that gravity works in your favour.

WEEK 21

HEARTBURN
What your doctor can do

Heartburn, an unpleasant burning sensation behind the breastbone, usually worsens as pregnancy progresses. You may also experience nausea and regurgitation of sour-tasting fluid in your mouth. If it becomes a severe or recurring problem that self-help measures do not alleviate, your doctor may first prescribe a low sodium antacid/alginate combination to relieve the symptoms. The latter coats the oesophagus and forms a 'raft' over the stomach contents, preventing them from coming back. You will be advised to use generous amounts after meals and before you go to bed. If the symptoms are very severe, your doctor may recommend one of the stronger acid suppressing drugs which may be safely used in later pregnancy.

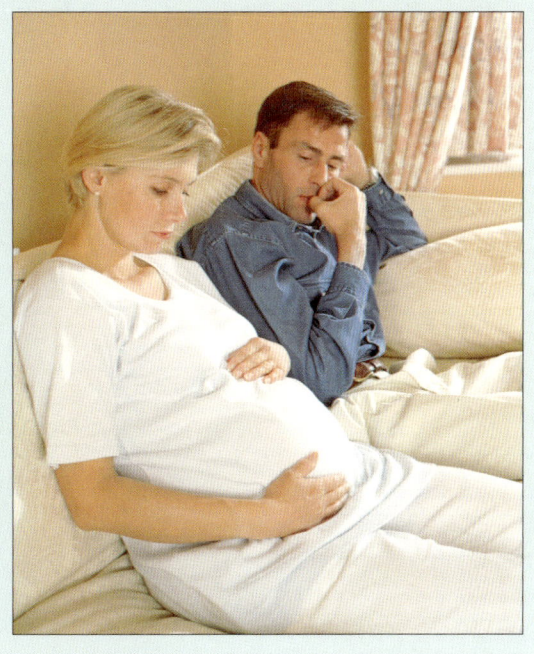

You are increasingly aware of your baby's different movements, and how he or she responds to outside stimuli, such as a loud noise or even the sun's warmth on your abdomen. You can feel the difference between when the baby is high up in your abdomen, or lying low in your pelvis.

What's happening to you

• You may be starting to experience heartburn after a large meal.

• You will be putting on weight at a rate of about 0.5kg (1lb) per week.

• As your uterus enlarges it will push up against your ribcage, and you may notice that your chest size continues to expand as your ribs spread out to make more room. You may need to adjust your bra to allow for this.

What's happening to your baby

• Your baby now weighs about 0.5kg (1lb), and is putting on more weight every day.

• Your baby moves freely, swimming around your womb – which can feel strange. He may even do the occasional somersault.

• Your baby lets you know he or she is there – the kicks and prods become stronger and more frequent as each week passes.

Avoid spicy foods

Although it is sometimes said that a good curry can help the onset of labour, spicy food can often aggravate heartburn. Try to avoid anything that might irritate your digestive tract, such as peppery, heavily spiced, very rich or very oily foods.

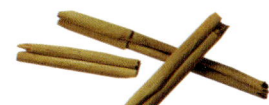

Very spicy food, such as Eastern cooking, can often play havoc with your digestion during pregnancy.

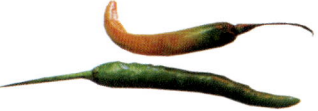

TWICE AS NICE

IF YOU ARE TOLD you are expecting twins, it can come as something of a surprise, particularly if there is no history of twins in your family. There's no reason to worry, but you will need to take extra care about the amount of rest you take and the food you eat, to prepare for the extra demands of carrying two babies.

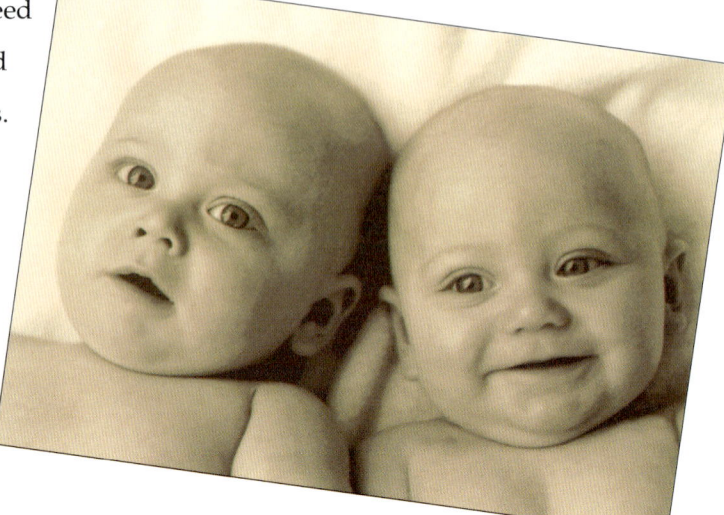

Women who are expecting twins usually find out during their first scan (16 to 18 weeks). However, as the babies at this stage are only half their eventual size, the view of one twin can sometimes be obscured by the other and so may not be visible in the scan. If there is some doubt, you will be asked back for a second scan in four or five week's time. Because there are two heartbeats, it is sometimes possible to detect the presence of twins by week eight.

A mixed blessing

It is understandable if some parents react to the news that they're expecting twins with a mixture of emotions. It can seem like a huge responsibility to have two babies to look after at the same time. But there is something magical about the relationship between twins that doesn't usually happen to the same extent between other siblings. As mum has two lives to nurture in her womb, she has some special requirements to help her and her growing babies through the pregnancy.

Take plenty of rest

Twins are harder work for mum to carry, so she needs to slow down and give her body a chance to cope with the extra load. If you are expecting twins, aim to have regular meals, regular rest times and go to bed early. Consider getting some extra help with the housework and shopping. Employed women expecting twins usually start maternity leave earlier (at about five months).

Eat well and wisely

Each twin often has a lower birthweight than a single baby. This is because there is less room in the uterus for twins, and they are often born at least three weeks before the usual term. So it is even more crucial that mother is well nourished.

The dietary advice given to all mums-to-be (see pages 20–23) needs to be modified for women who are expecting twins. They need more iron (from meat, fish, spinach and dried fruit), calcium (five daily servings of low-fat dairy products) and lots of folate-rich foods (such as leafy green vegetables, wheatgerm, pulses and fortified breakfast cereals).

Have regular check-ups

Women carrying twins are more prone to pregnancy problems. These include oedema, pre-eclampsia, nausea, tiredness and anaemia (a low red blood cell count, usually due to iron deficiency). Twin-mums are usually called in for check-ups more often, and may be offered more frequent ultrasound scans. Labour is always monitored in hospital as there are special risks related to delivering twins.

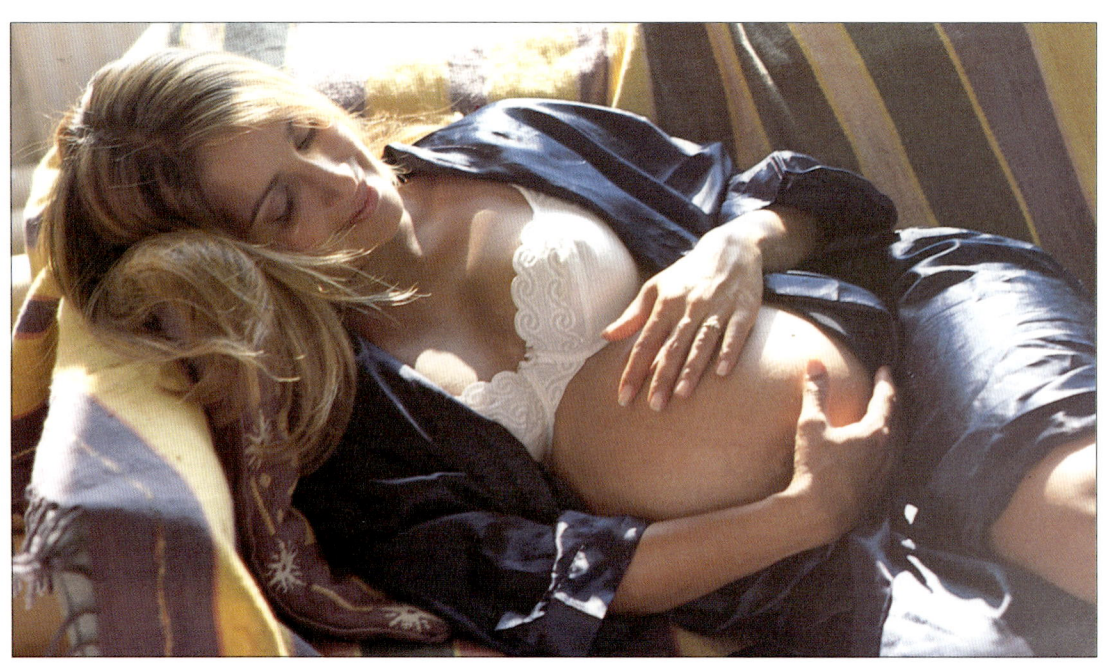

TWIN TYPES

Make mine a double

There are two main types of twin: fraternal and identical. Which type occurs is determined by events either before conception or after implantation in the uterus.

Fraternal Twins

Most twins are fraternal. They are conceived when two eggs are released from the ovary at the same time and are fertilised by separate sperm. Both fertilised eggs travel down the uterine tubes in the normal way, and both successfully adhere to the side of the uterus. They develop independently within separate amniotic sacs. They both have their own umbilical cord attached to their own placenta. As the eggs and sperm that produced them had different genetic codes, the two babies are not identical, and may even be different sexes.

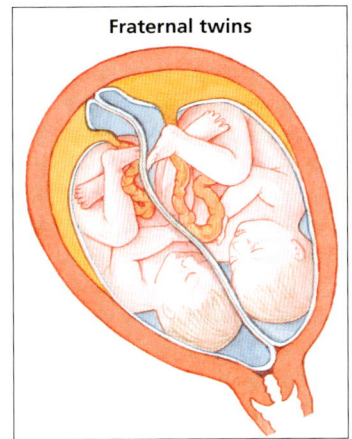

Fraternal twins

Fraternal twins develop when two eggs are fertilised simultaneously. They have their own placentas and umbilical cords.

Identical Twins

Identical twins

Identical twins. Much rarer, and occurs when one egg is fertilised, which then splits. They can share a placenta, but usually have their own umbilical cords.

In three out of ten conceptions that result in twins, only one egg is released, which is fertilised by one of the partner's sperm, but then for some reason divides to produce identical twins. This division usually occurs after the fertilised egg has attached itself to the uterine wall. As a result, identical twins usually share the same placenta but have their own umbilical cords. If the egg divides early, the twins may have separate placentas and separate amniotic sacs. These babies share the same genetic code and are always the same sex. Although identical twins look very similar, and other people find it difficult to tell them apart, they still have their own very individual personalities.

FACT BOX

Twins are more likely than single babies to be born by Caesarean section. Nevertheless, around 75 per cent of twins are still delivered vaginally.

The birth of twins

Having a twin birth is more difficult than a singleton birth. All are managed in hospital as care must be taken with the extra risks associated with twin deliveries, such as a longer wait for the second twin who has to let his sibling go first, or a lower than average birth weight. Many midwives recommend forceps or a Caesarean section if the time interval between the births is longer than 15 or 20 minutes.

Cephalic twins

Breech/Cephalic twins

Above: In a breech/cephalic presentation, one twin lies bottom down, and the other is head down.

Left: In a cephalic presentation, both twins lie head down.

During your antenatal visit, you will be measured with a tape from your sternum to the top of your pelvis, usually by the midwife. Don't worry unduly if you are told that you are 'small for your size'. Many women have a relatively small abdomen at this stage in their pregnancy, especially if they have a small build or less amniotic fluid surrounding their baby.

What's happening to you
• You may get a stitch down your side more often. This is sometimes caused by the muscles in your side stretching to accommodate your new shape.

What's happening to your baby
• Your baby's fingernails are starting to grow, as are the lines on the palms of the hands. The patterns that these lines make are unique and will stay the same throughout your baby's life.
• Your baby's arms and body are much more in scale with the head. These proportions will now remain until birth.

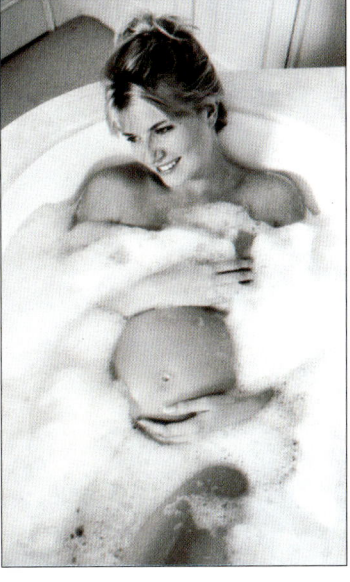

• Your baby is often much more active when you are resting.

YOUR LOVE LIFE

COUPLES OFTEN find that this is a special time in their relationship as their sexual needs adapt to meet the challenges of pregnancy. Provided your partner is gentle, and there are no special considerations with your pregnancy that make intercourse inadvisable, there is no reason why you should not continue to enjoy a satisfactory and fulfilling sex life.

The physical changes you are going through at this time and the effects of the pregnancy hormones on your body may alter your attitude to sex and the way your body responds to arousal. Every woman's experience is different and there is no way of predicting how it is going to be for you. Any time from the second trimester onwards, many women find that they become more interested in sex, and more easily aroused.

The symptoms often experienced during the early months, such as fatigue and nausea, which can put a woman's sex life on hold for a while, may now no longer be a problem. Indeed, you may be discovering that your natural energy levels and desires are beginning to return to normal.

Alternatively, you may find that you remain less interested in sex right through your pregnancy and after your baby is born. This is a perfectly natural response, and you should not let it upset you or your partner.

Changing responses

Blood flow to your breasts and genitals has now greatly increased to help facilitate the physical changes of pregnancy. This also causes these areas to respond more quickly and more fully to stimulation and, in particular, to become more aroused and swollen during sex. In particular, your vagina and clitoris will be more sensitive, and your vaginal secretions will increase, making penetration easier and more pleasurable for both of you. You may also find that you experience orgasms more easily and more intensely.

Intercourse will not usually hurt your baby. The amniotic fluid that surrounds the baby provides an effective cushion against bumps and bruising. As you get bigger, however, it may be wise to avoid positions that involve your partner's weight pressing down on your abdomen. There are alternative positions you can use such as side-by-side or 'spoons'.

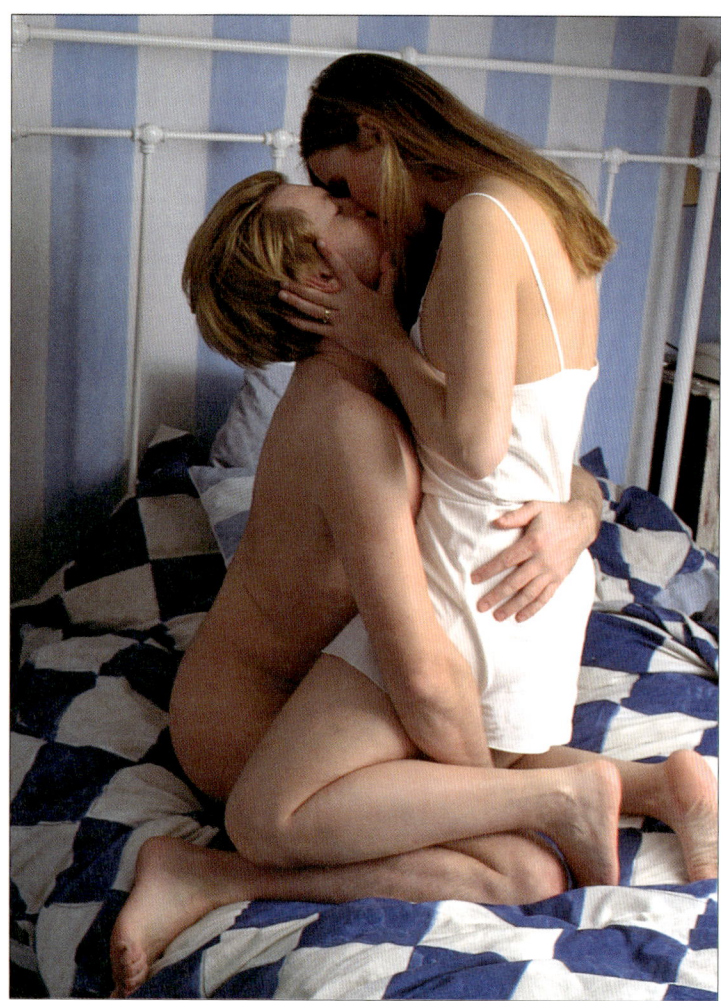

PREGNANCY POSITIONS
Sexual Alternatives

As you get bigger you may find that it is more comfortable to adopt a sexual position that does not put pressure on your abdomen.

• Side-by-side position, with the man and woman lying facing each other, is ideal for tender, unhurried lovemaking.

• Spoons position, so-called because the couple seem to fit together like two spoons, is similar to side-by-side except that the man enters his partner from behind.

• Woman-on-top position allows the woman to control the depth of penetration, and she feels more supported.

• Rear entry is a less satisfactory position in pregnancy as the woman needs to support herself on her hands and knees in order to keep their combined weight off her abdomen. The woman may also find that it puts excess strain on her back. The man can enter very deeply at this angle, so unless he is very careful this can be uncomfortable for the woman.

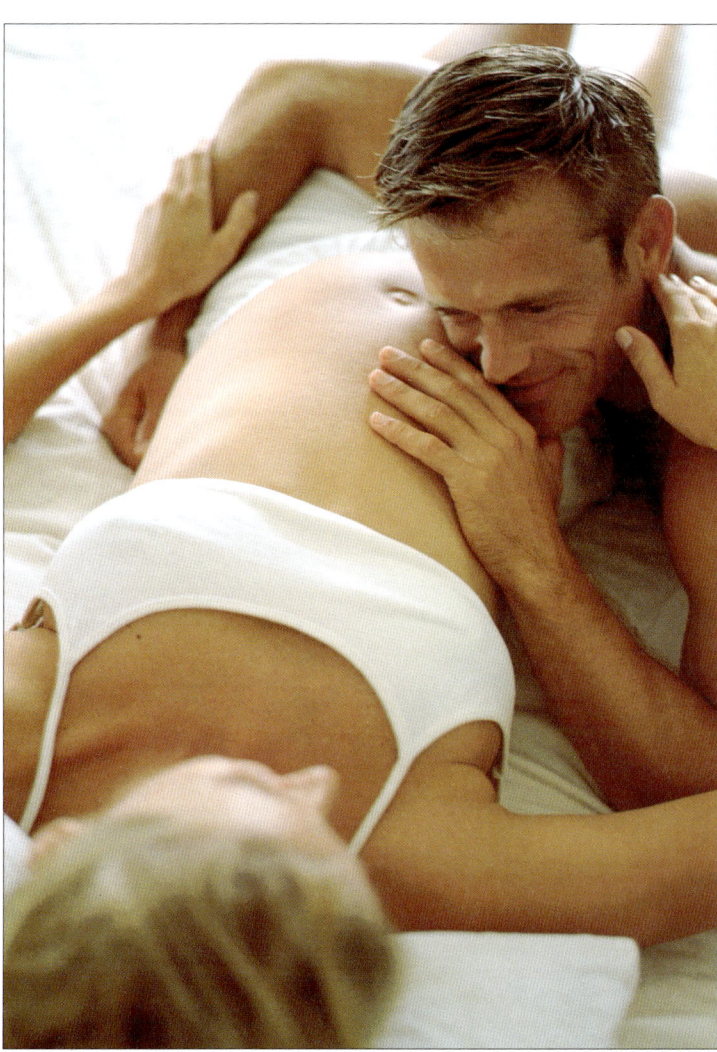

WEEK 23

Your midwife will be able to identify the different parts of your baby's body through your abdomen just by touch. This form of physical examination is called 'palpating'. It allows the midwife to determine the size, position and direction in which your baby is lying in the uterus.

What's happening to you

• You may start to feel what seem like contractions, but this does not mean you are going to give birth prematurely. They are called Braxton Hicks' contractions and are a form of 'rehearsal' for the muscular movements that will occur during labour.

What's happening to your baby

• Your baby can hear your voice, and will respond to your words, so you can now start to bond with your baby.

• Your baby can also hear and recognise your partner's voice, and studies have shown that fathers who speak to their unborn child are able to bond more quickly.

• If a suitable piece of soothing music (nothing too rousing) is played repeatedly while your baby is in the womb, he or she will respond to it and will be calmed by it after the birth.

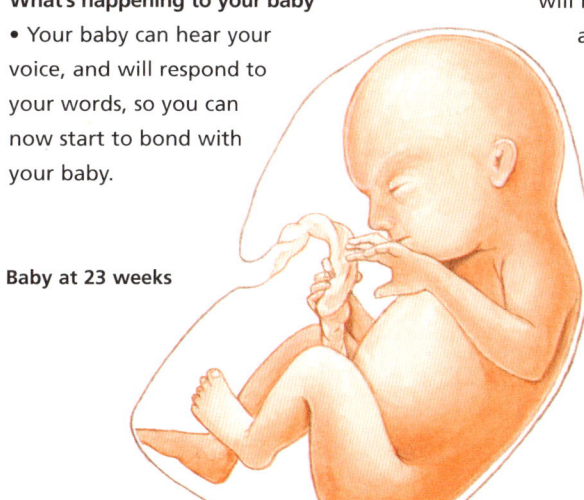

Baby at 23 weeks

It is also advisable to refrain from very athletic sex. Although this is not necessarily dangerous, it may cause you some discomfort. You may find that your breasts and nipples are very tender at times, and may need to ask your partner to be a little more gentle.

Some women are advised to refrain from intercourse during their pregnancy. This is more likely if a woman has experienced some bleeding, or if she is expecting a multiple birth, as the doctor may be concerned about the risk of miscarriage or premature labour. But there are many other ways of sharing physical affection with your partner, such as oral sex or mutual masturbation. Just spending

time touching and stroking each other or giving each other a massage, can be a deeply sensual experience.

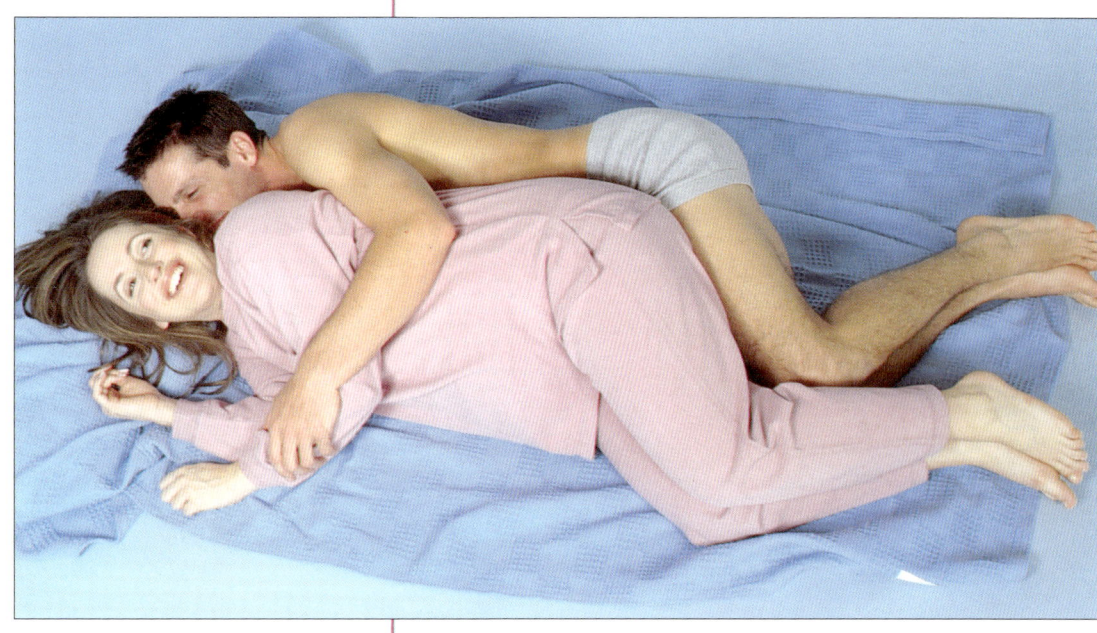

YOUR PELVIC FLOOR

A GROUP OF muscles and ligaments at the base of the abdomen, known as the pelvic floor, plays a key role during pregnancy and labour. If you practise a few simple exercises every day to tone and strengthen these structures you may have a more comfortable pregnancy, an easier delivery and a much lower risk of postnatal complications.

The pelvic floor supports all the major organs in the pelvic region, including the bladder, rectum, uterus and vagina. A woman's health and comfort are greatly influenced by this group of muscles and ligaments and their ability to do their job. The pelvic floor is under greatest strain during pregnancy. The added weight of the fetus, uterus and amniotic fluid place a heavy burden on the pelvic floor and can lead to weakening.

Aid to childbirth

Strong pelvic floor muscles are particularly important during labour as they help you to bear down and push as you give birth to your baby. It is also important to have a strong pelvic floor after the birth, when your body returns to its pre-pregnancy condition. You can strengthen and tone your pelvic floor by doing the exercises described on these pages every day.

The stronger the pelvic floor muscles remain during pregnancy, the quicker they will recover afterwards. It usually takes about three months for full recovery following delivery.

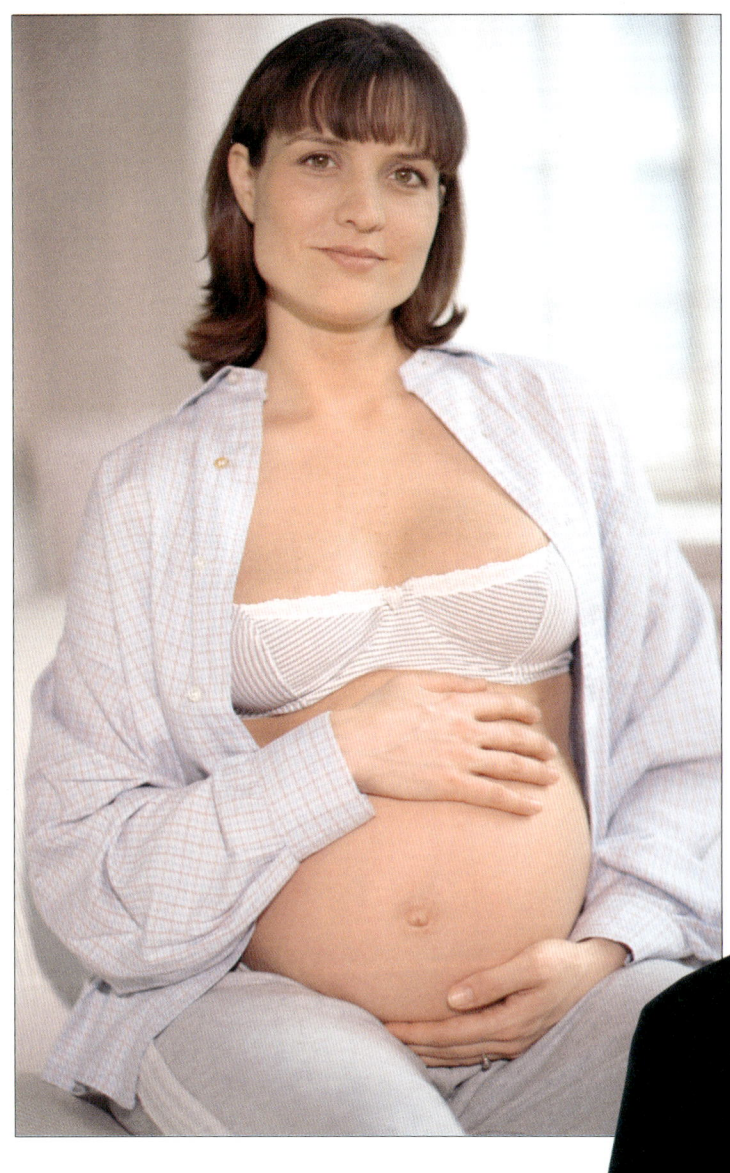

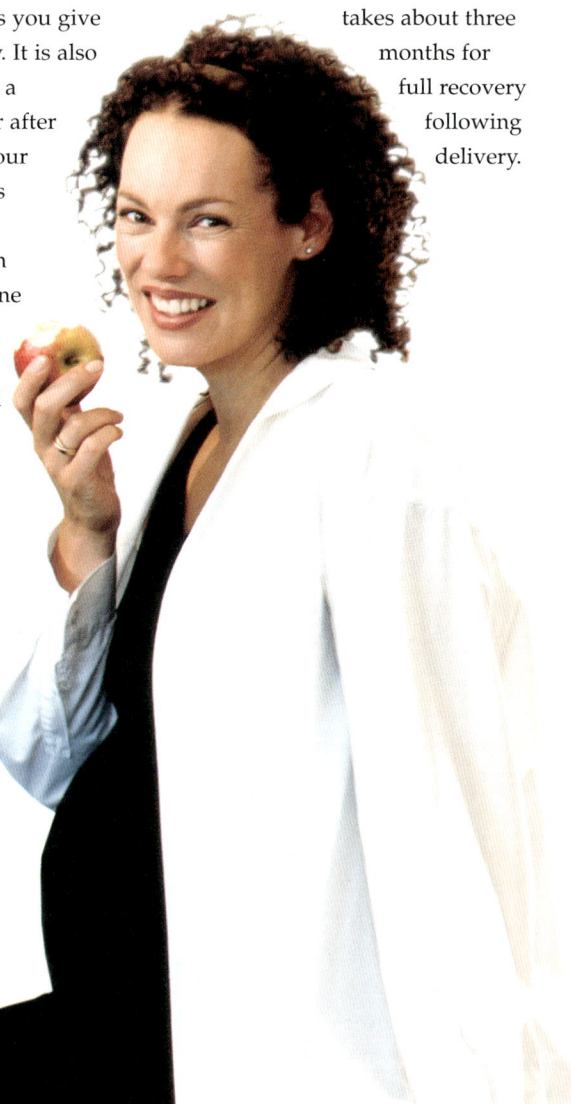

Having a strong pelvic floor can also reduce the risk of serious complications, such as uterine prolapse. This is when the uterus drops down slightly from its usual position into the vagina.

By strengthening your pelvic floor you can also improve your sex life. The more firmly you squeeze your pelvic muscles during intercourse, the more pleasurable it is for you and your partner.

During the later stages of your pregnancy, you may find that you experience a slight leakage of urine, especially when you sneeze, cough, laugh or walk up stairs too quickly. This is an indication that the pelvic floor is being placed under increased strain and is unable to fully control your bladder as it used to.

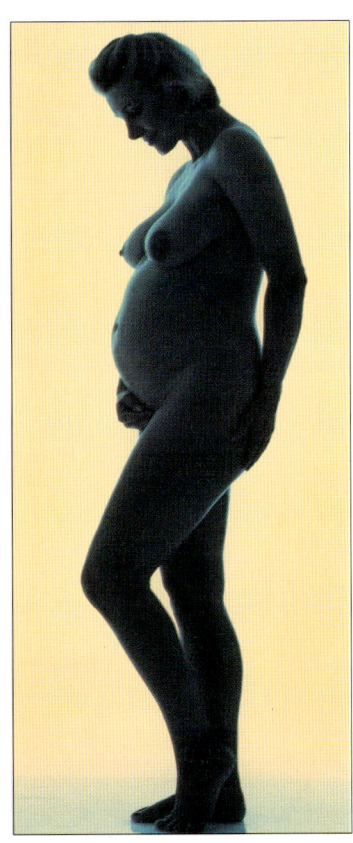

PELVIC FLOOR
Exercises for muscle tone

Performing these exercises every day can help you to maintain the strength and tone of your pelvic floor muscles. You can exercise your pelvic floor whenever you remember, sitting, standing or lying down, at work or at home, as no one else will know what you are doing – and you don't have to go to the gym. Aim to do the following routine six times a day – it is very quick and easy.

1 Sit upright in a comfortable chair and relax. Try to 'isolate' the pelvic floor muscles by concentrating on them as you relax the rest of your body. To identify your pelvic floor muscles, imagine you are urinating and trying to stop the flow. You will feel a tightening in your anus, vagina and bladder. The muscles you use to do this make up your pelvic floor.

2 Tense the muscles, and try to hold for a count of ten, and then release them slowly. Repeat this tensing and releasing action five to ten times, breathing normally as you do so. You will find this becomes easier to perform the more you practise. Do ten quick tense-and-release cycles, without holding for a count. This will help your muscle tone.

WEEK 24

If you are worried about your rise in weight, remember that a major part of this increase is due to your developing baby. If you are worried about losing your figure, tell yourself it is only temporary, and by following a healthy diet (pages 20–23), and taking regular exercise (pages 28–31), your body will resume its pre-pregnancy state quite quickly after the birth.

What's happening to you
• The top of your uterus can be felt above your navel.
• You will be feeling your baby kick all the time now, and may be keeping a kick chart. Don't let this slide – it is important to monitor your baby's activity in the womb as this is another indication that your pregnancy is proceeding well.

What's happening to your baby
• Your baby's heartbeat can be heard by means of a fetal stethoscope placed on your abdomen, which your midwife will sometimes use. A heartbeat of about 160 beats per minute is an indication of good fetal health.
• Your baby's lungs are developing well, as more air sacs form inside the lungs every day. The nostrils are open and the diaphragm moves up and down as the baby's chest expands. This gives your baby a chance to practise breathing before the birth, when he or she will have to start breathing air for the first time. Until babies are born they actually take small amounts of fluid in and out of the lungs.

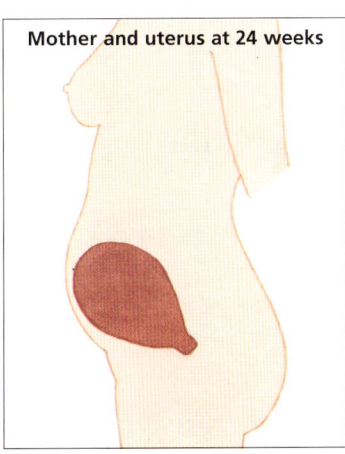
Mother and uterus at 24 weeks

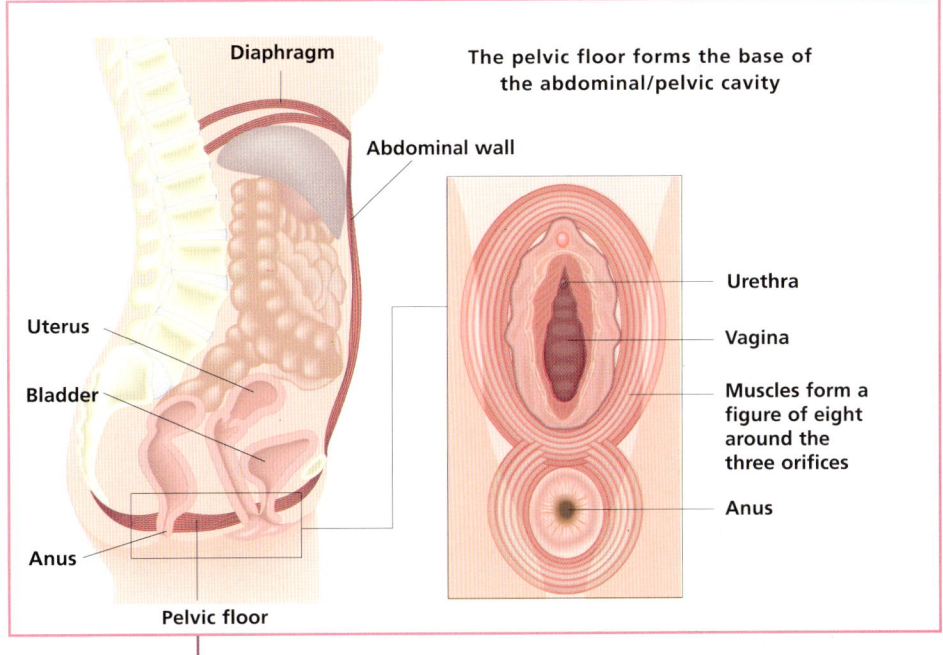

Diaphragm

The pelvic floor forms the base of the abdominal/pelvic cavity

Abdominal wall

Uterus

Bladder

Anus

Pelvic floor

Urethra

Vagina

Muscles form a figure of eight around the three orifices

Anus

SEEING RED

VAGINAL BLEEDING during pregnancy is more common than many people think. It does not necessarily mean that something is seriously wrong with you or your baby. However, if you do become aware of any abnormal bleeding it is advisable to consult your doctor, and note any other signs or symptoms that might help to identify the cause.

We tend to associate abnormal vaginal bleeding during pregnancy with miscarriage. In fact, pregnancy is a complicated process, and there are many reasons why bleeding can occur. The cause usually depends on whether you are at an early or late stage in your pregnancy.

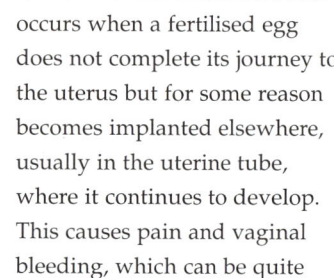

For example, it is fairly common for your first missed period to be marked by some light 'spotting', but this rarely indicates that anything is wrong.

Early pregnancy

ECTOPIC PREGNANCY: This occurs when a fertilised egg does not complete its journey to the uterus but for some reason becomes implanted elsewhere, usually in the uterine tube, where it continues to develop. This causes pain and vaginal bleeding, which can be quite severe. The pregnancy has no chance of continuing to term and the woman may require emergency medical treatment. Ectopic pregnancy is potentially very dangerous, so you should contact your doctor at once if you experience abdominal pain and vaginal bleeding early in pregnancy.

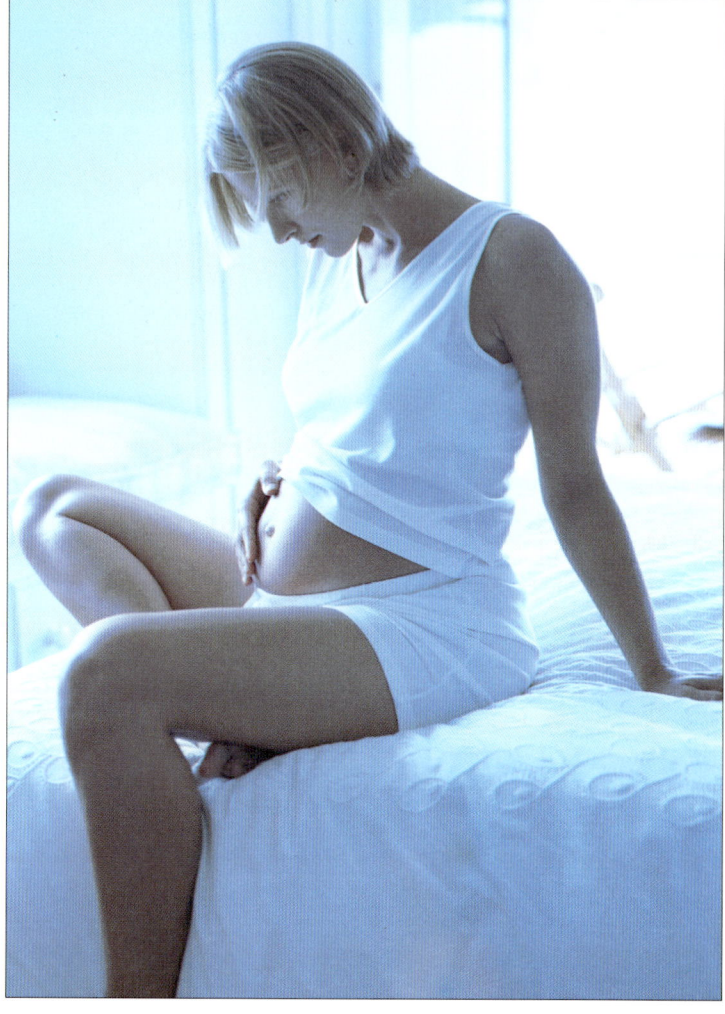

MISCARRIAGE: If termination of a pregnancy occurs before 24 weeks, it is termed a miscarriage; after this date it is referred to as a stillbirth. Miscarriage in the early months is often the result of an abnormality in the embryo. It may be the body's way of rejecting an embryo that would not survive anyway. It can also be caused by severe illness in the mother, or an abnormality in her uterus, such as fibroid growths. Sometimes the endometrium is not thick enough to enable the embryo to become attached, or to obtain sufficient nourishment.

Late pregnancy

PLACENTAL ABRUPTION: In this condition, part or all of a normally situated placenta comes away from the lining of the uterus. It can be caused by injury, or placenta praevia (see opposite) but often occurs for no known reason. It is more common in women who have had several children. Bleeding can be accompanied by pain, tenderness or a tightening sensation in the uterus or abdomen, or aching in the lower back. In some cases there is no bleeding. The condition can be mild to severe, depending on the

MEDICAL ADVICE BY DR. CAROL COOPER

VAGINAL BLEEDING
When there is no cause for alarm

Vaginal bleeding during pregnancy is alarming but some causes are innocuous. However, always seek medical advice if you notice abnormal bleeding.

- When the fertilised egg attaches to the wall of your uterus, there may be implantation bleeding. This is sometimes taken as a light period.
- Occasionally, there is slight bleeding when a period would have occurred for the first few months of pregnancy.
- Cervical erosion (a velvety patch on the cervix) or a polyp (a grape like swelling on a stalk) can produce a little spotting, which is often worse after intercourse.
- Varicose veins may occur on the cervix, vulva and in the vagina and may cause bleeding.
- Bleeding from piles or from the urinary tract may be confused with vaginal bleeding.

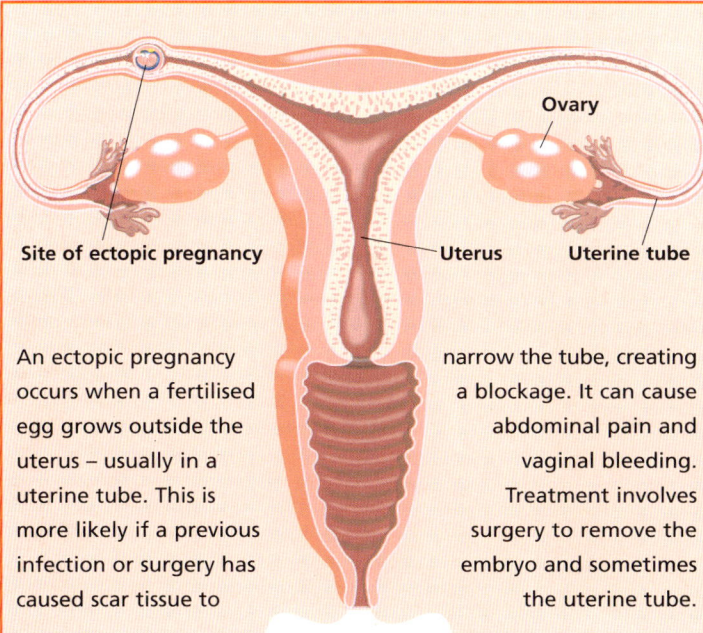

Ovary

Site of ectopic pregnancy   Uterus   Uterine tube

An ectopic pregnancy occurs when a fertilised egg grows outside the uterus – usually in a uterine tube. This is more likely if a previous infection or surgery has caused scar tissue to

narrow the tube, creating a blockage. It can cause abdominal pain and vaginal bleeding. Treatment involves surgery to remove the embryo and sometimes the uterine tube.

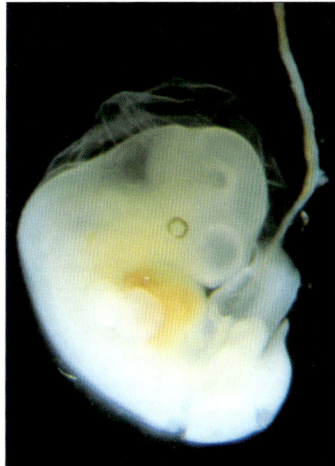

An ectopic pregnancy can be dangerous for the mother and requires immediate medical attention. Instead of travelling to the uterus, the embryo develops in the uterine tube, causing pain and bleeding.

amount of bleeding and the area of the placenta that has become detached. In mild cases, where light blood loss is experienced and less than one quarter of the placenta has separated, bed rest is usually advised and the pregnancy has a good chance of continuing to term.

PLACENTA PRAEVIA: In some women, the placenta becomes attached to the uterine wall in an abnormally low position. Bleeding occurs because the lower part of the uterus grows fastest in the later stages of pregnancy, causing part of the placenta to become detached

from the uterine wall. If the placenta covers the cervix, vaginal birth will not usually be possible, and the baby will be delivered by Caesarean section. The cause of this condition is not known, although it is more common in women who have had several children.

This week marks the end of your second trimester – you are two-thirds of the way through your pregnancy. This can be a frustrating time when many mums say they are 'just waiting around for the birth'. Try to be patient. Your body will initiate labour when you and your baby are ready. Although your baby is now fully formed, every day spent in the womb is precious as he or she puts on extra weight and gathers strength for life on the outside.

What's happening to you
- You may be getting leg cramps.
- You find you need to urinate even more often as your growing baby and expanding uterus press on your bladder. There's not much you can do to prevent this, but pelvic floor exercises will help bladder control (see pages 54 and 55) and so are worth doing for this reason alone. The problem will stop once the baby is born.

What's happening to your baby
- Your baby's brain is growing to fill the skull, which is now in proportion to the rest of the body. The neural connections multiply as the brain matures, enabling signals from the brain to travel down nerve fibres and activate the muscles.
- As your baby's blood circulation gets stronger and fat builds up under the skin, he or she begins to develop independent temperature control.
- The marrow in your baby's bones is now producing red blood cells which are circulating in the bloodstream.

SKIN CARE

YOUR SKIN undergoes various changes during pregnancy, mainly due to your expanding waistline and the hormones circulating around your body. If you are going to develop skin conditions such as stretch marks and dry, oily or itchy skin, they will have appeared by now. Don't worry, there are ways to help your body cope with these problems.

The physical changes to your body that occur during pregnancy not only have a fundamental effect on your appearance but can also profoundly effect the way you feel. It is impossible to predict exactly how each individual will be affected by the physical and chemical changes that pregnancy brings about, but knowing what to expect and learning how to help your body adapt can go a long way to maintaining your sense of wellbeing.

Stretch to fit

Ninety per cent of pregnancies leave stretch marks, with varying degrees of intensity. They are most likely to appear as roughly parallel, curved lines across the abdomen – the area that expands most during pregnancy. Some women also experience minor stretch marks on other areas of the body, such as the thighs and hips, and sometimes even the breasts and upper arms.

The marks may appear very noticeable at first – reddish marks on white skin, or white marks on skin with a darker pigmentation. As your skin adapts, however, especially once the pregnancy is over, they will fade to softer marks that are far less noticeable.

The causes

Stretch marks are caused by two main factors. The pregnancy hormones in your body tend to break down some of the fibres in your skin, which makes it less flexible and also causes the change in colour. The skin is then stretched by your expanding abdomen, and is unable to revert to normal once the pregnancy is over.

Unfortunately, there is nothing you can do to prevent stretch marks entirely. But you can reduce the problem by taking care to keep your skin as supple and flexible as possible, for example by regular use of skin creams, oils or moisturisers after you bathe.

Itchy skin

You may find that your skin becomes very itchy, particularly in hot weather. This is partly due to the increased blood volume circulating around your body, which raises your temperature and causes you to perspire more freely, resulting in

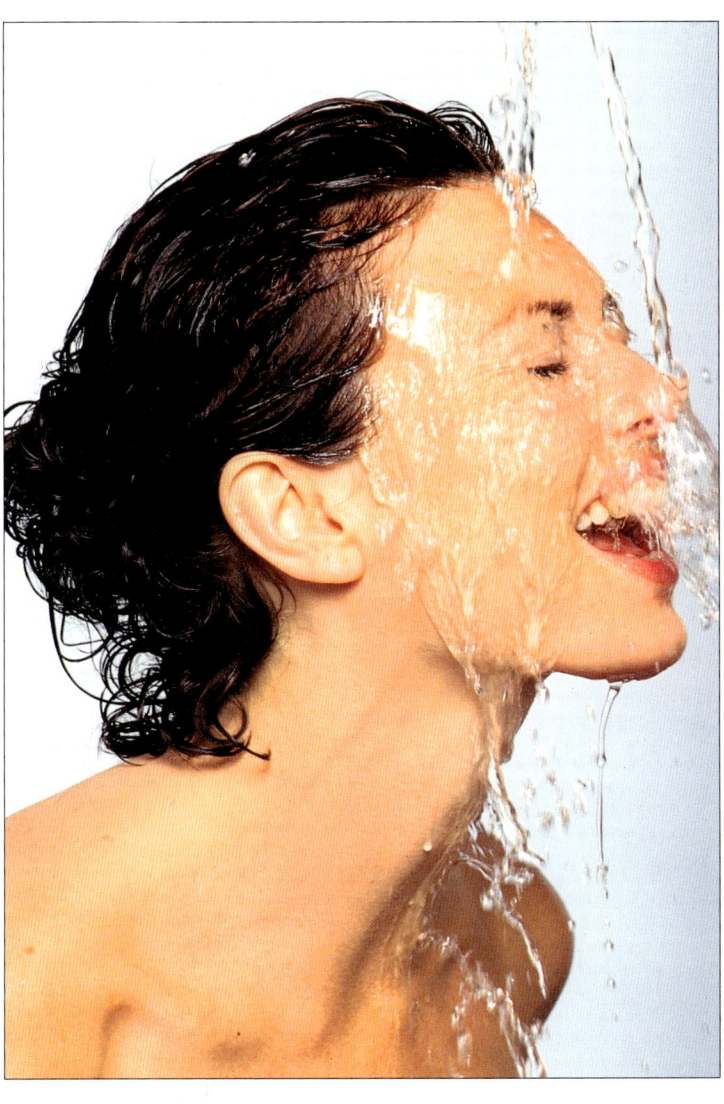

sticky, uncomfortable skin. You will notice the itchiness most around your thighs and abdomen, especially where the skin is being stretched most, and the skin between your thighs may chafe and become sore. Again, this problem tends to be worse in hot weather when you perspire more.

To help reduce this problem, wear only natural fabrics, which are more effective than man-made fibres at allowing the skin to breathe. You should also wear loose-fitting clothes as much as possible to allow the air to circulate around your body and to prevent the material rubbing against your skin.

Calamine lotion can help relieve the itching, redness and soreness, and skincare oils and creams rubbed into problem areas will keep the skin lubricated and supple and help prevent chafing. If the itching becomes very severe, you should tell your doctor or midwife as, in rare cases, it may indicate a more serious medical problem.

SKIN REMEDIES
Keep your skin well oiled

• Ordinary soap can remove the oils in your skin that keep it supple, leading to dry inflamed skin. Choose a moisturising or oil-based soap to help replace these natural oils.

• Bath oils help reverse the dehydrating effects of bathing. Remember that you should never have the bath water too hot as this can harm your baby, who cannot regulate body temperature as easily as you can.

• Aromatherapy oils, such as lavender or camomile, can be helpful. Add a few drops to a gentle massage oil, such as sweet almond, and apply after a bath or before bed, whenever the itching is persistent. Just rubbing something into your skin helps.

• Makeup can help by boosting your confidence, especially when you are feeling tired and think that you are not looking your best.

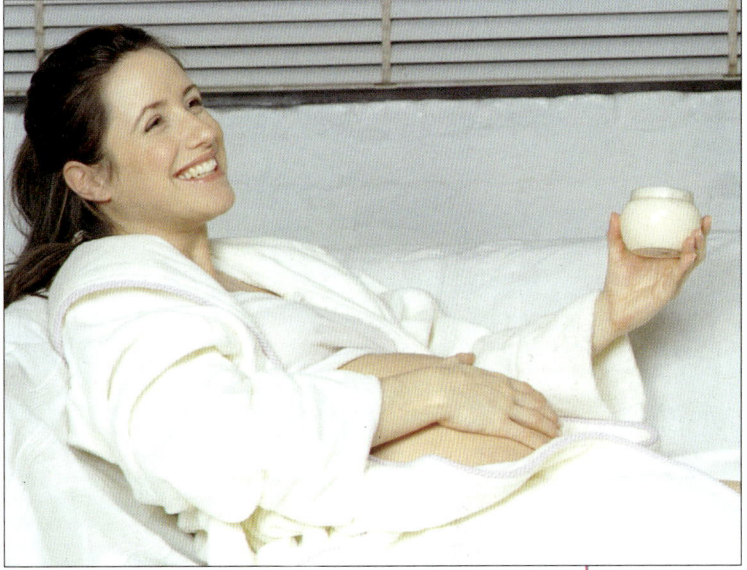
Skin creams will help with itchiness, and may reduce stretch marks.

WEEK 26

By now your breasts have reached an advanced stage in their preparations to breastfeed your newborn. A thick, yellowish fluid called colostrum will already have formed in readiness to feed your baby for the first few days. Colostrum is lower in fat and sugar than breast milk but higher in protein and minerals.

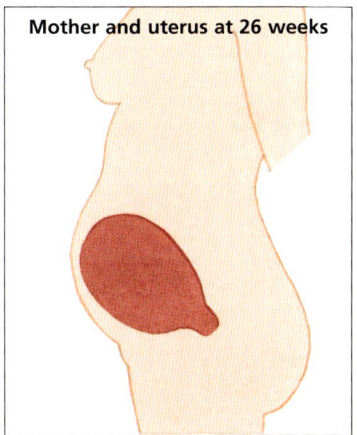
Mother and uterus at 26 weeks

What's happening to you
• Stretch marks may start to appear around your hips and abdomen, if they haven't already.

What's happening to your baby
• Your baby's skin is becoming thicker, with more layers of fat forming just under the surface to provide insulation.
• Your baby's skin is becoming more opaque. The fine network of veins and blood vessels lying just beneath the surface are no longer visible.

HELLO IN THERE!

YOUR BABY hears every sound in the outside world that is loud enough to reach the uterus. Your baby also hears you when you speak – and has started to bond even before the birth. You can make use of this early opportunity to communicate with your baby to help form a rapport that can last a lifetime.

Studies have shown time and again that mothers who talk to their baby in the womb and pat him or her through their abdomen are rewarded with an infant that is happier, puts on weight faster and is more responsive to her calming words. Fathers who take an active role during pregnancy and start relating to their new baby before the birth are also able to form a closer bond. This is a chance to get to know your baby from the very beginning.

Your baby is aware

It may be that mothers who are more inclined to stroke and talk to their baby in the womb are simply more in tune with their baby's feelings, and therefore better able to respond to the infant's emotional needs. Nonetheless, an unborn baby does have a memory, and can see, hear and feel much of what is going on in the world outside the uterus wall. So it makes sense that relating to your baby early on will be of great benefit after the birth.

Your heartbeat is a constant companion to your baby as he or she grows inside you, and when you speak, your baby will be able to hear what you say, although it may sound slightly muffled. If dad wants to talk to your baby, ask him to place his mouth close to your abdomen and speak quietly. Unborn babies prefer calm, relaxing noises, much as they prefer their mums to move in a gentle way. They don't like sudden, jerky movements, or booming noises, and will become distressed by them. You should always bear this sensitivity in mind and try to moderate your actions as much as possible.

A world of sound

As your baby has an active memory, any piece of music that you play to calm your baby in the womb can also be used to soothe your baby after he or she is born. It has been shown that slow, simple melodies such as lullabies tend to work best.

Curiously, the sound of a hairdryer has also been found to have a calming effect on a newborn baby. This is thought to be because it sounds similar to the 'whooshing' sound of mother's blood moving around her body that the baby hears in the womb.

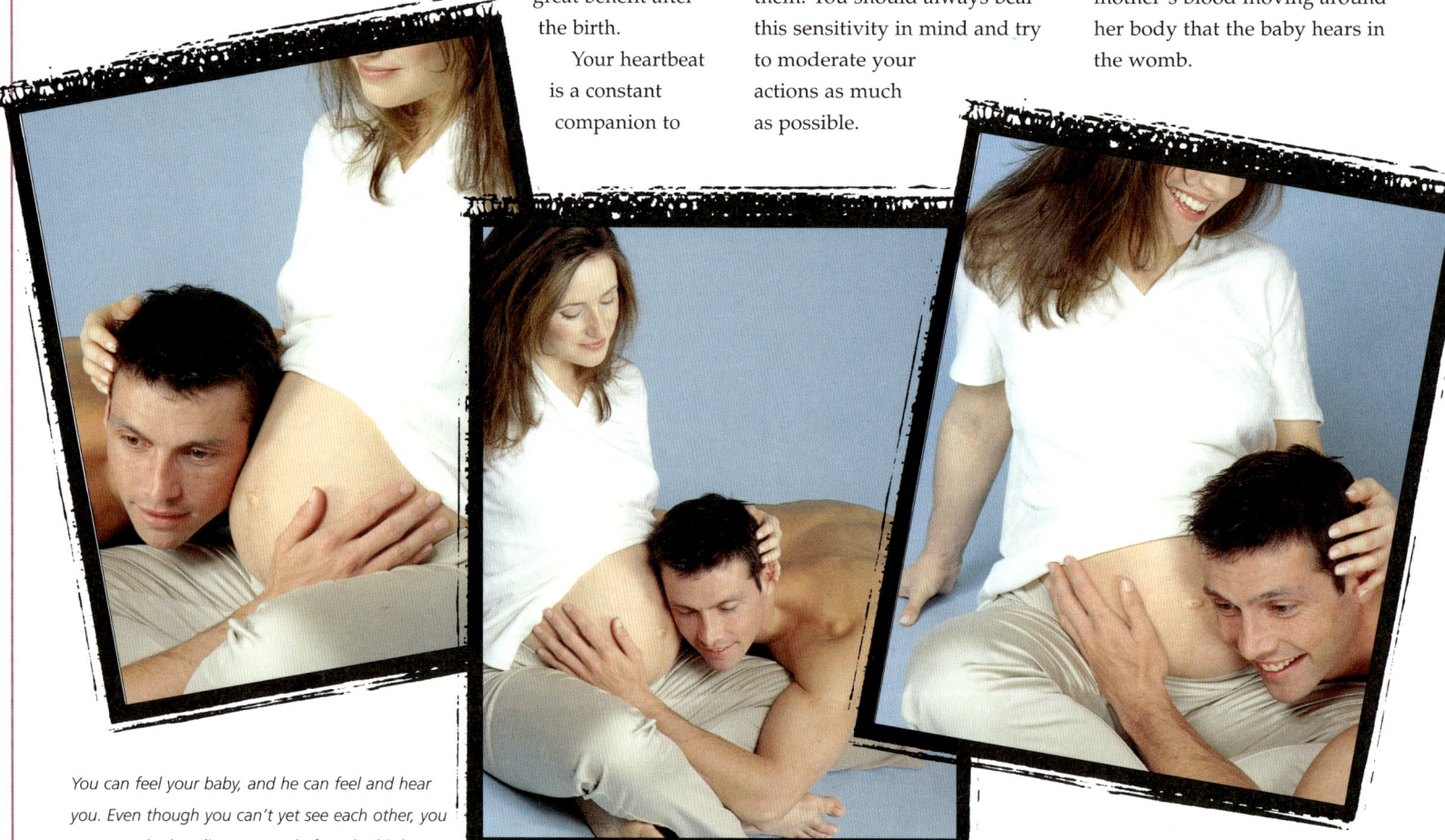

You can feel your baby, and he can feel and hear you. Even though you can't yet see each other, you can start the bonding process before the birth.

WEEK 27

Your bump is noticeable even through your clothing, and you may find that complete strangers offer you their seats on public transport, or let you go to the front of queues. Accept their assistance with good grace. Don't feel that they are belittling you in some way, most people are simply aware that pregnancy is a demanding and tiring time for mum.

What's happening to you

• You will find that you have to visit the lavatory more often than before. As the space inside you gets more cramped, there is simply less room for your bladder to expand, so it has to be emptied more often. This will get worse in the last month – at about week 36 – but you'll be pleased to know it immediately returns to normal after delivery.

• You may start to have trouble sleeping, if you haven't already. Your increasing size makes it more difficult to find comfortable positions, and your nocturnal lavatory visits are more frequent. Your baby may occasionally be more active than usual, which can also add to the problem of restless nights. Do try to get as much sleep as possible – your baby is still growing at a rapid rate and needs you to be as rested as possible.

Baby at 27 weeks

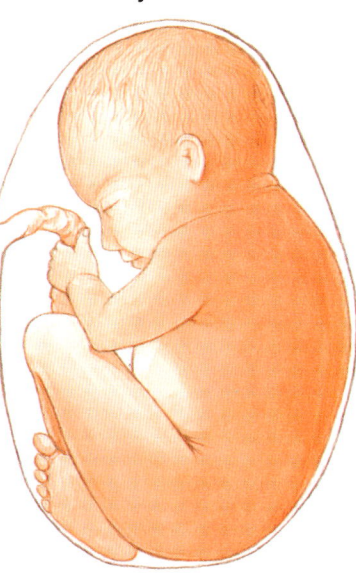

Shared emotions

If you get angry, sad, frightened or excited your baby will feel the same emotions. This is not because your baby knows what you are thinking, but because the chemicals released into your bloodstream (such as adrenaline or endorphins) cross the placental bridge and enter your baby's bloodstream. This happens within seconds. If you find yourself becoming stressed, tense or anxious, the best thing to do is to try to be calm, and to soothe your baby with gentle words and stroking actions. Your baby will hear your voice and feel your hand, and be comforted by your attentions.

What's happening to your baby

• Your baby now weighs just over 1kg (2^1/$_2$lb) and is 26cm (10^1/$_2$in) from crown to rump.

• Your baby's nervous system is still developing: the brain grows larger still, and increasing numbers of connections are being made between brain cells and nerves.

• Your baby's delicate eyes can now open, as the protective covers have fallen away, so he or she can practise blinking and looking around.

• Your baby's kicks will feel stronger but he or she is much more cramped in your uterus, and can no longer swim about or do somersaults as before.

TESTING, TESTING

FACT BOX

Having a baby today is statistically safer than it has ever been, during both pregnancy and delivery.

DURING PREGNANCY, your midwife and doctor will perform what can seem like a bewildering array of tests to check that you and your baby are well. Many of these tests, such as blood and urine, are routine, but in some cases there may be a need for more specialised screening techniques.

Routine blood tests carried out during pregnancy can sometimes indicate a possible abnormality in the fetus. One of the tests carried out analyses levels of alphafetoprotein (AFP), a chemical initially produced by the embryo's yolk sac and later on by the fetal liver. Abnormal levels of this chemical might indicate developmental disorders such as spina bifida or hydrocephalus (excess fluid inside the skull), or a chromosomal disorder such as Down's syndrome.

Specialised tests

An abnormal result is not conclusive, and can often turn out to be a false alarm, or an abnormality that is so minor it is not worth worrying about. Where possible, an ultrasound scan will be used to check whether or not there is a problem. In some cases, however, the mother may be offered more specialised tests. This is more likely if there is an increased risk of abnormality, perhaps because there is a

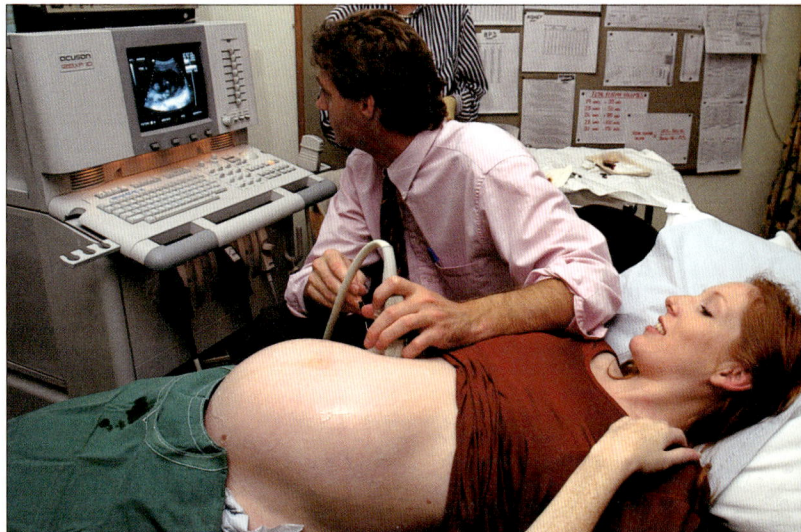

history of genetic disorders in the woman's family or that of her partner.

The risk of having a Down's syndrome baby increases with age. If your baby is at risk from Down's syndrome you may be offered the 'triple test', which measures levels of AFP along with other hormones found in a pregnant woman's blood. However, the triple test is not conclusive – it can only indicate the level of risk.

In order to confirm a genetic disorder or Down's syndrome, the mother may be offered a screening test such as amniocentesis or chorionic villus sampling. It is up to you whether or not you wish to take

Ultrasound is one of the most common 'windows to the womb', and has revolutionised antenatal care.

The image on the screen may look confusing at first, but the operator will point out the main features.

testing further and obtain conclusive evidence regarding such abnormalities. Your doctor will explain the procedure and risks in detail and answer any other questions you may have.

Amniocentesis

This test can be carried out to diagnose Down's syndrome and genetic disorders. During amniocentesis, a doctor gently inserts a needle through the woman's abdomen into her uterus to draw off a small amount of amniotic fluid. An ultrasound scanner is used to guide the needle and ensure there is no damage to the placenta or fetus.

Amniotic fluid contains cells from the baby which can be

MEDICAL ADVICE BY DR. CAROL COOPER

GENETIC PROBLEMS

What are your choices?

If your baby has a serious genetic abnormality confirmed by amniocentesis, your obstetrician will discuss your options with you. Essentially, these are either to allow the pregnancy to continue or to terminate it. No decision can be made without your consent. You may be referred to a genetic counsellor who will explain the implications for any future pregnancies. It may be possible to meet and talk to parents who have had a similarly affected child. Take your time, and try to get all the facts and opinions before deciding. If you decide to continue your pregnancy, you will need to prepare yourself emotionally for the birth of your child and the problems that may follow.

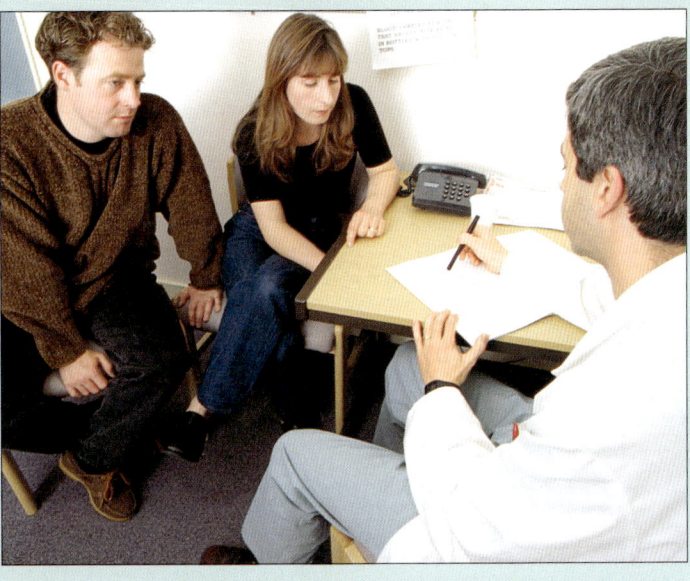

Your obstetrician will discuss your choices with you both, should a fetal abnormality be identified during any antenatal testing. Consider your options carefully.

Support from your partner, family and friends is invaluable throughout, whichever course you choose to take.

Your midwife will now be taking particular note of your baby's orientation, and especially the direction in which the head is facing. The information is needed in planning for the delivery as certain positions (like the 'breech' position where the baby wants to come out bottom first) can make for a more difficult birth.

What's happening to you

• Back pain can be an increasing problem as the greater weight you are carrying affects your walking posture. Try to safeguard your back as much as possible by paying attention to your posture when you are sitting and walking (see pages 68 and 69). Take frequent rests and prop a small cushion into the small of your back. Avoid wearing high-heeled shoes which push your pelvis forwards and put extra strain on your lower back.

What's happening to your baby

• As the free space inside the uterus steadily diminishes, so your baby will start to settle into a head-down position in the next four weeks or so in preparation for delivery.

grown (cultured) in a laboratory and analysed to reveal the baby's genetic or chromosomal makeup. The test is usually carried out between weeks 15 and 17 and the results take up to three weeks to come through. There is a slight risk involved, a small proportion (under one per cent) of amniocentesis tests result in miscarriage.

Chorionic villus sampling

CVS is a newer test and offers an alternative to amniocentesis. It gives similar information about the baby's genetic and chromosomal makeup.

To carry out chorionic villus sampling, a small tube is passed through the vagina or abdomen to take some finger-like scraps of tissue called chorionic villi from the placenta.

This procedure carries a slightly higher risk of miscarriage

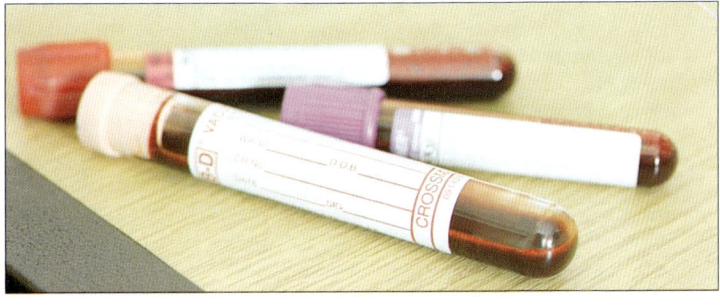

Blood tests (above) are carried out during pregnancy, and an amniocentesis test (right) may offer peace of mind.

(around one per cent), but can be performed earlier (any time after 10 weeks) and the results are usually available within two weeks (and sometimes in days). This is much faster than amniocentesis. This means that if a problem is found and a decision is taken to terminate the pregnancy, an abortion can be carried out at an earlier and safer stage.

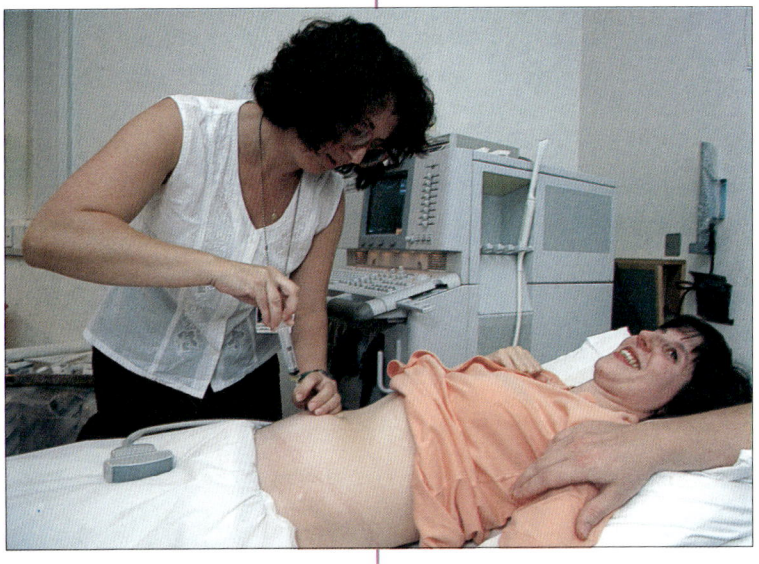

IN THE BLOOD

ONE RARE complication of some pregnancies occurs when the mother's blood type is incompatible with that of her baby. The blood test that is carried out early on in all pregnancies should alert doctors to such a problem so that the necessary measures can be taken to ensure the health and safety of the child.

FACT BOX

A baby's blood type is inherited from one of the parents. For an Rh-negative woman to have an Rh-positive baby, her partner must be Rh-positive too.

All blood is categorised as either Rhesus (Rh) positive or Rhesus negative. Part of all routine blood testing in the early stages of pregnancy is to check the Rhesus status of the mother. Rh-negative blood is relatively rare – only 15 per cent of all mothers have this blood type. Their pregnancies will need to be monitored in a special way as complications can arise if their baby is Rh positive, but provided the pregnancy and delivery are managed properly all should be well.

Risk to baby

If the mother's blood is Rh negative, it is tested every two to three weeks to check for the presence of antibodies. These are the agents in the mother's blood that fight against any foreign body – including Rh-

positive blood cells. These antibodies would attack the baby's blood, thereby putting the unborn infant at risk.

Antibodies are produced in an Rh-negative mother's bloodstream in response to any Rh-positive blood cells that may be introduced, a process called sensitisation. In the past, this most often occurred when the woman gave birth to an Rh-positive baby. Although the first baby is usually unaffected, the antibodies produced then attack subsequent Rh-positive babies. Doctors now take steps to prevent this happening. Sensitisation may also occur during any invasive antenatal testing (such as amniocentesis), or as a result of a miscarriage, or termination, or if haemorrhaging occurs during the pregnancy.

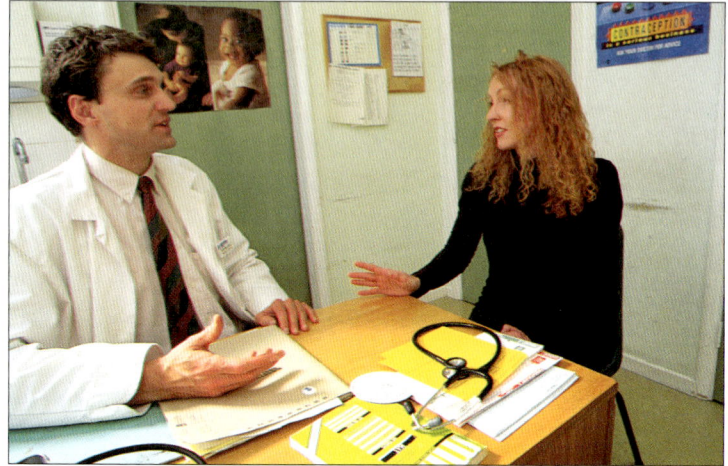
Your specialist will explain your choices and the testing procedures available to you.

Checking the baby

If antibodies are detected in an Rh-negative woman, the doctor may want to monitor the health of the growing baby. This can be done with an ultrasound scan at 18 weeks, or with a cordocentesis. Here a needle is inserted into the umbilical cord to take a

blood sample. The procedure is much like an amniocentesis but the sample is of fetal blood and not amniotic fluid.

If the fetus is found to be anaemic (that is, has a low red blood cell count) it may be because the baby's blood is being attacked by the mother's

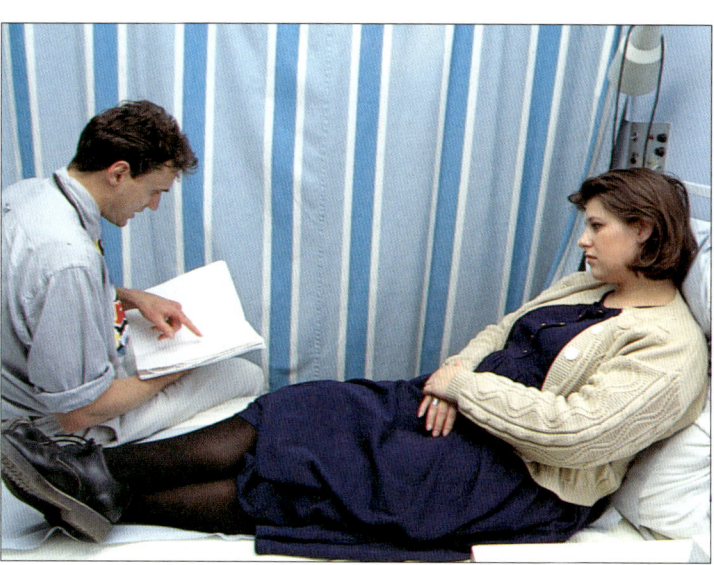
Before any hospital testing, the nurse and doctor will go over your notes with you.

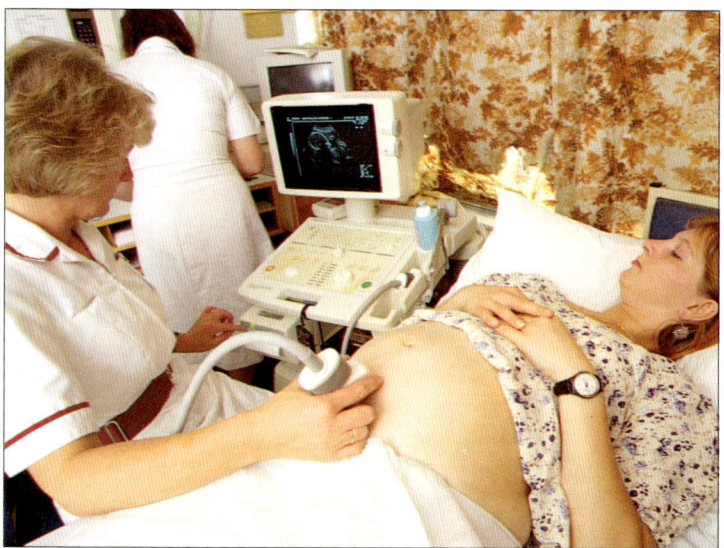
Ultrasound is used in a lot of antenatal testing procedures as it is safe and non-invasive.

WEEK 29

MEDICAL ADVICE BY DR. CAROL COOPER

LIFE-SAVING INJECTIONS
Rhogham jabs

The antiserum jabs given to Rh-negative mothers carrying Rh-positive babies are known as Rhogham injections. The women are injected up to 48 hours after they give birth to their first baby, or after a miscarriage, termination, amniocentesis, or any form of haemorrhaging. The injection is designed to prevent the production of antibodies.

If the woman does not receive this injection and once again carries an Rh-positive baby, the antibodies present in her blood may cross the placental barrier and attack the red blood cells of her baby.

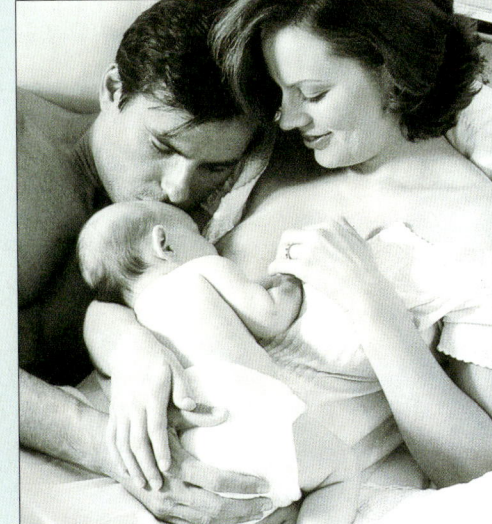

antibodies, in which case further steps will need to be taken. In extreme cases, if the baby is far enough advanced, the birth may be induced early so that a blood transfusion can be given to completely rid the baby's blood system of the mother's antibodies. This is not an option doctors take lightly, as it is safer for babies to continue to develop inside their mother's uterus – a far better environment than a hospital's premature baby ward.

Today, health professionals are aware of the problem of rhesus incompatibility and routinely administer an antiserum injection to counter the production of harmful antibodies. As a result, complications arising from an Rh-negative mother carrying an Rh-positive baby are becoming increasingly rare.

You will definitely notice your baby's stronger movements and hearty kicking. This helps to develop the infant's muscle tone. Your baby can see, and so is aware of light and dark, but the field of vision is limited to 20cm (8in) – about as far as there is to see inside you. Even after your baby is born, he or she can still only see this far, but the infant's vision rapidly develops to cope with longer distances and brighter and more vibrant colours.

What's happening to you

• You may find you suffer cramp more often, in which case increasing your intake of reduced-fat dairy foods may help.

• Colostrum may occasionally leak from your nipples. This is perfectly normal, but to protect your nipples from getting sore you might consider buying breast pads. These are round, absorbent disposable pads for pregnant and nursing mothers to help keep the nipples dry – constant dampness is one of the main reasons for chafing and soreness. Nipples can crack and bleed during breastfeeding, so it is worth starting to take good care of your breasts from now on.

What's happening to your baby

• Your baby is 26cm (10½in) from crown to rump and weighs nearly 1.5kg (3lb). The size of your baby's head is now in correct proportion to the limbs.

• The fatty deposits under your baby's skin are continuing to build up, with the result that the skin now looks less wrinkled and more like that of a plump newborn baby.

• Your baby is now breathing in a regular way, and the air sacs inside the lungs continue to develop, although they are protected by a special fluid in the womb.

FACT BOX
You may need to buy bigger shoes now as many women find their feet swell by as much as half a size during the last few months of pregnancy.

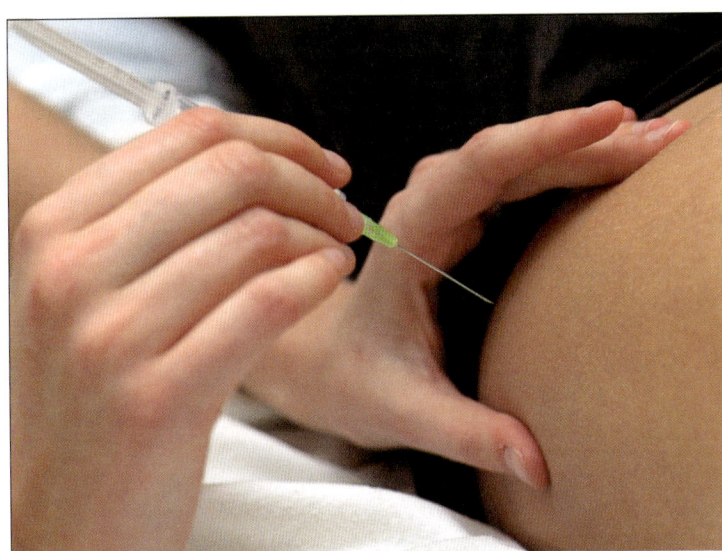

Rhogham injections will prevent harm to future babies of Rhesus-negative mothers.

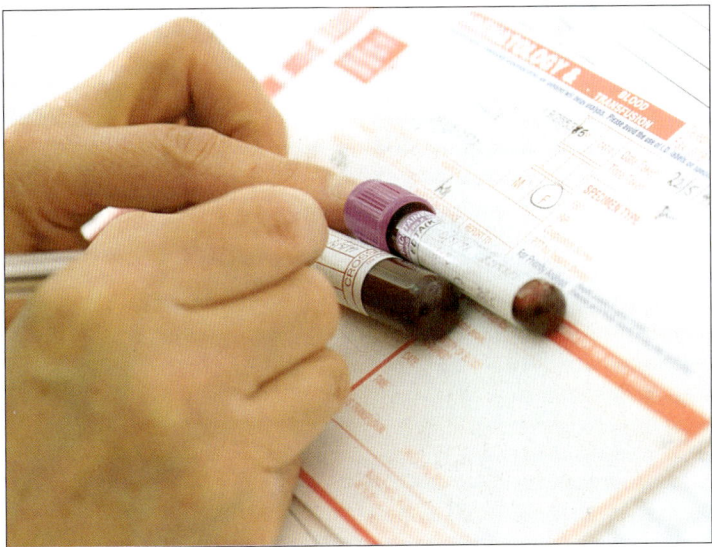

Blood testing is common in every pregnancy to provide detailed medical information.

SHOPPING FOR BABY

IT IS NEVER too early to think about clothing and equipment for the new baby. There is a bewildering choice of 'must-have' items available to new mothers, so if you're not careful the cost can quickly mount up. With careful planning and bargain-hunting, however, you can cut the effort and expense involved.

FACT BOX On average, parents spend £2,000 (US $3,250) on baby equipment in the first year.

You should start collecting all the necessary clothing and equipment for your baby's first months well before the birth. You'll need most of these things almost immediately, and you probably won't have much time to go shopping after the baby is born. A new baby quickly outgrows clothes so, to keep costs down, take advantage of any offers of second-hand items from other mums whose babies no longer need them.

Essential items

The range and number of items you buy will largely be determined by the cash you have available. But there is a minimum number of essential items, so draw up a list of the most important things to help you keep within your budget. If friends and family want to contribute, you could give them a copy of the list, or mention the items you have yet to obtain.

Cot

For the first few months, your baby will happily sleep in a carrycot or Moses basket, but will then need a proper cot or crib with bars. Make sure the gaps between the bars are no more than 6cm (2½ in) wide, and that the mattress is washable. Choose one with a drop side to reduce back strain. Some cots

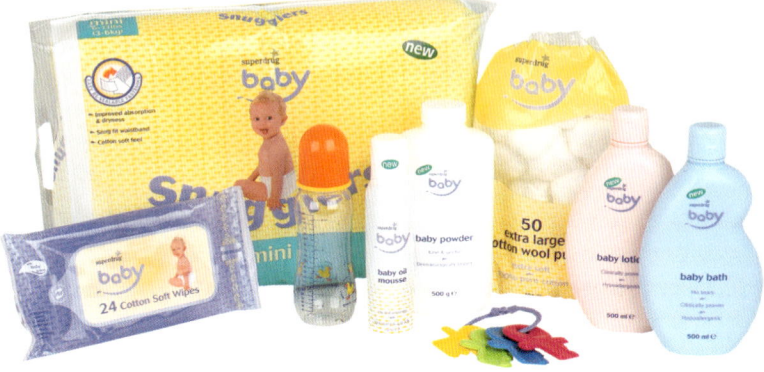

Prepare for your new arrival with a selection of babycare products – it makes a lot of sense to buy these necessities early.

convert into a child's bed, which saves money later on. Avoid using a duvet or cot bumper during the first year as they can cause overheating, a possible contributing factor in cot death.

Changing Area

You will need to set aside an area for bathing and changing baby. You could use a chest of drawers, with a soft wipeable changing mat on top, and buy a baby bath to place inside your bathtub. Alternatively, buy a dedicated changing table, usually with a bath fitted into it. Whatever you use, make sure it is waist high, to reduce bending and lifting and so ease the strain on your back (but never leave your baby unattended on a raised surface because of the risk of falling).

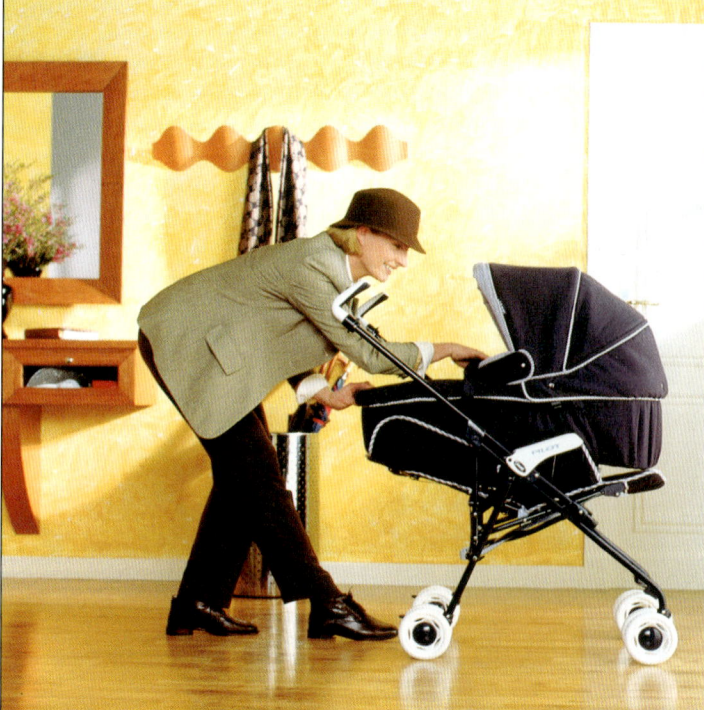

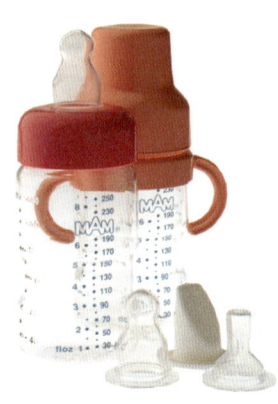

Above: Baby rockers are really useful accessories for newborns.

Left: You will need a pram – probably one of your biggest early expenses.

Right: Don't forget bottles and teats, even if you are planning to breastfeed.

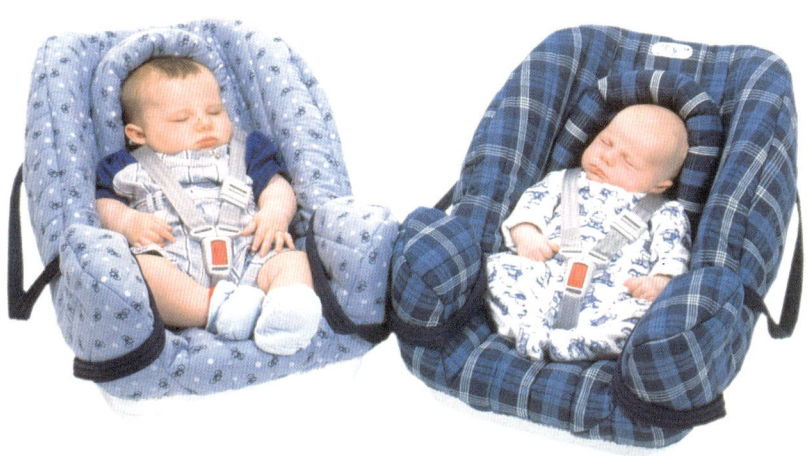

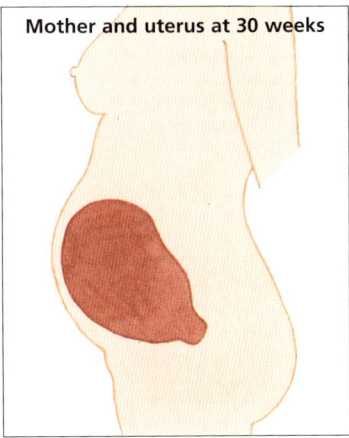

FACT BOX

The nursery should be well ventilated but free from draughts – a temperature of 18–20°C (65–68°F) is ideal.

WEEK 30

Storage

You'll need a place to store nappies, wipes, cotton balls (for wiping and cleaning), nappy rash cream, muslin cloths (for wiping up regurgitated milk), and soft towels to dry the baby.

Linen

Choose soft cotton blankets, which will not irritate the skin or cause overheating, unlike wool or man-made fibres. Closely woven kinds are best, so the baby's fingers can't get trapped in the holes. Avoid ones with long fringes, which might choke the baby.

Nappies

If you are using terry nappies, you'll need a storage bucket to keep them in until they can be washed, plenty of nappy pins, and nappy liners. It is a good idea to get a packet of disposables as well (the smallest size available), in case you need to change the baby in a hurry.

Clothing

Colour and style is a matter of personal preference – your baby will only be interested in comfort – but value for money and practicality are also important considerations. Cotton is best next to the body, as it will not irritate the baby's delicate skin. You will need: vests, knitted tops, socks, all-in-one stretch suits, mittens, hat and shawl.

Pram or Pushchair

There is a bewildering array of prams and pushchairs available, so choose one to suit your purse and your needs. It should fold up to a convenient size and shape without too much fiddling. For car users, a pram with collapsible frame may be best; if you use public transport, a pushchair that folds horizontally is ideal. It should have a carrycot or sturdy seat that lies flat (your newborn won't be able to sit up for at least five months) but also converts into a forward- or rear-facing seat. The brakes must work without your needing to hold on to the handle.

Car Seat

For safety's sake – and by law – all infants and children in cars must be carried in a securely fitted car seat or cot. Some types (called 'travel systems') are specifically designed to take cots and prams. They require less strapping and unstrapping, and allow a sleeping baby to be moved without being disturbed.

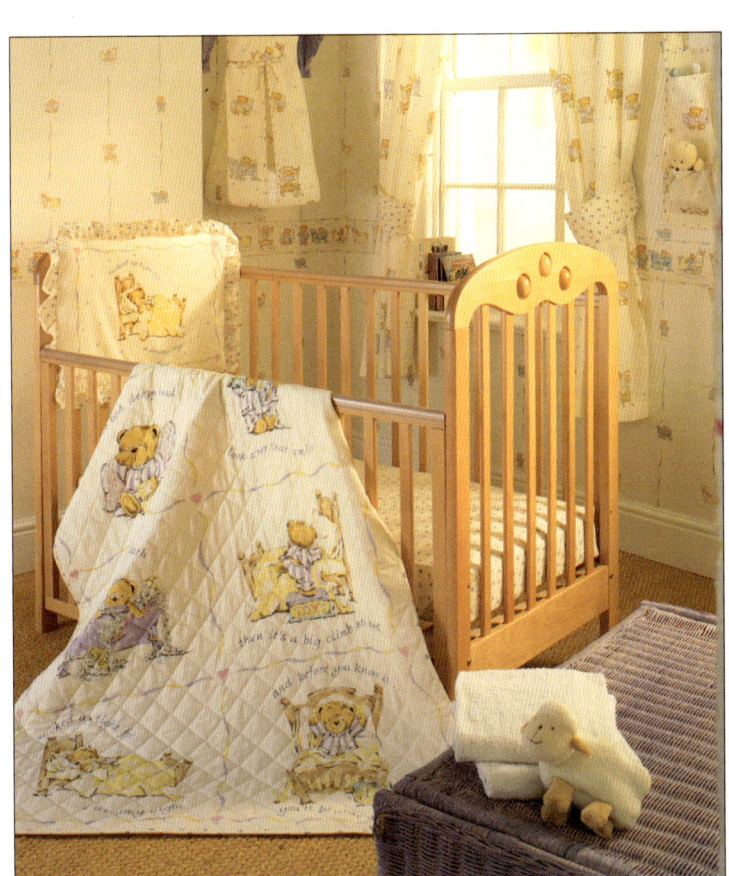

Get your nursery ready well in advance. The last thing you will have time to do with a newborn baby is redecorate.

You may be feeling a little 'off-balance' because of the weight of the baby. This can take time getting used to, and many women remain a little unsteady on their feet until after their baby is born. Your baby has developed to such an extent that almost all babies born after 30 weeks survive.

Mother and uterus at 30 weeks

What's happening to you
• Your expanding uterus is reducing the space inside you still further and your ribs may now feel a little sore.
• Your pelvis is widening, which may also cause some soreness.
• The line down the centre of your abdomen (the linea nigra) may appear very dark now.

What's happening to your baby
• Braxton Hicks' contractions may last up to half a minute by this stage and your baby is aware of them, even if you can't feel them most of the time.
• Due to the increasing fatty layer under the baby's skin, he or she is now a healthy pink, rather than a reddish colour.
• Your baby is still coated with protective vernix and may even be born with this covering, which easily washes off.

TAKE IT EASY

YOUR BABY is putting on weight at a faster rate every day, with the result that your body is now under even greater strain and you are feeling increasingly tired. It is more important than ever that you pay attention to good posture, take extra care when moving around and rest whenever you can.

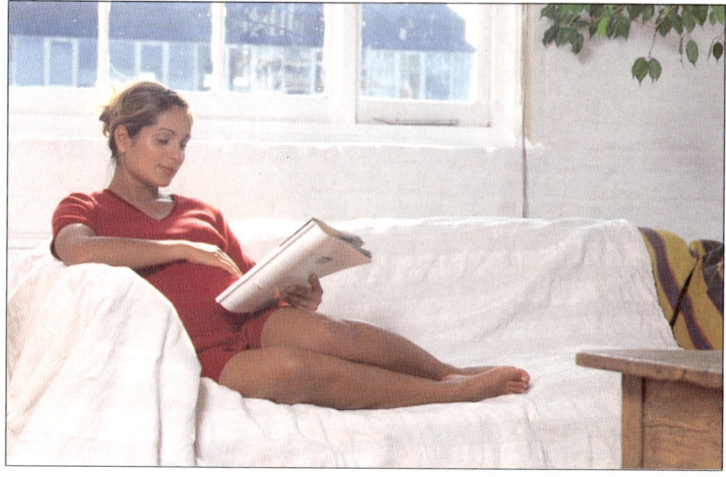

The added weight you are carrying is putting extra strain on areas of the body such as the spine and legs. This is not only a burden, but is also located in an area where you are unused to carrying heavy loads, placing an unusual strain on muscles and ligaments. It also alters your weight distribution, making it harder to balance.

Injury risks

These factors are not only very tiring but also increase the risk of injury, especially when combined with hormonal changes. The pregnancy hormone relaxin, which softens the pelvic ligaments to make childbirth easier, also slackens other ligaments, weakening the back and joints. You can reduce the risk of injury by taking some simple precautions.

LIFTING: The lower part of your spine is under greatest strain during pregnancy. Avoid any heavy lifting and be careful even with items you would normally consider within your capabilities. Keep your back straight, and never lean forwards or backwards when lifting. This ensures that your legs take most of the weight – they have the strongest muscles in the body.

Consider making more frequent, but lighter, shopping trips, in order to reduce individual loads. If possible, ask a shop assistant or companion to load your bags and carry them to the car or bus, and ask your partner or relatives to fetch bulky items for you.

POSTURE: Avoid sitting in one position for too long. You may find it more comfortable to rest in a semi-kneeling position while holding a bean bag or other large cushion as a support for your abdomen. Lying flat on your back can cause dizziness, especially in later weeks. You may find you'll sleep more comfortably lying on your side. Place pillows around you to support your abdomen and legs.

Leg problems

Swollen ankles, caused by oedema, or fluid retention, can be an increasing problem. Some women also develop varicose (swollen) veins caused by blood collecting in the legs. This is because the veins are under greater pressure during pregnancy and less efficient at squeezing blood back to the heart. Oedema and varicose veins can be very uncomfortable and may be made worse by standing for long periods, waiting in a queue, for example.

Putting your feet up, literally, for part of every day helps in several ways. By elevating your legs, you reduce swelling, and aid blood flow back to the heart, easing varicose veins. You are also getting a rest and taking the strain off your back. Never sit with your legs crossed, however, as it impedes blood flow and increases the risk of thrombosis.

The right touch

Getting your partner or a friend to massage your neck and shoulders gently can really go a long way to easing any built up tension during pregnancy. It also helps your baby as the resulting endorphins will enter the fetal bloodstream through the placenta, and produce a feeling of wellbeing.

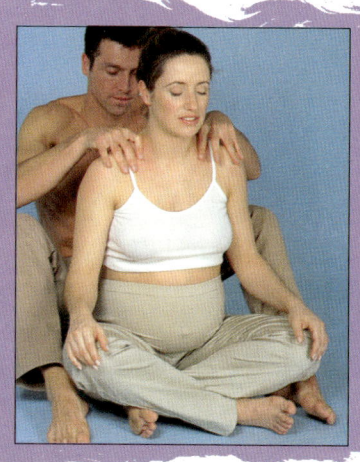
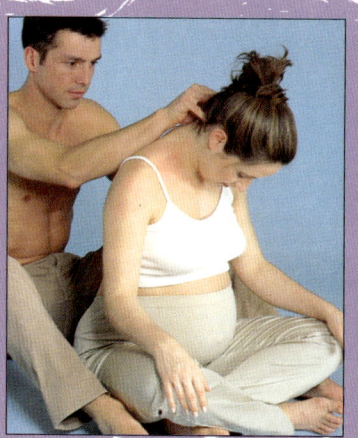
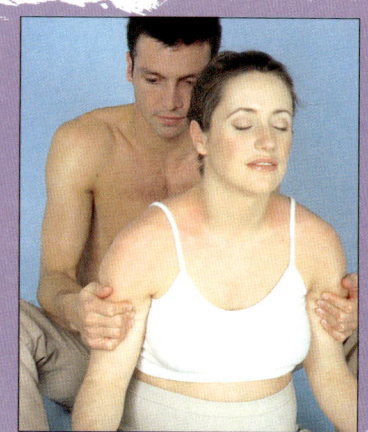

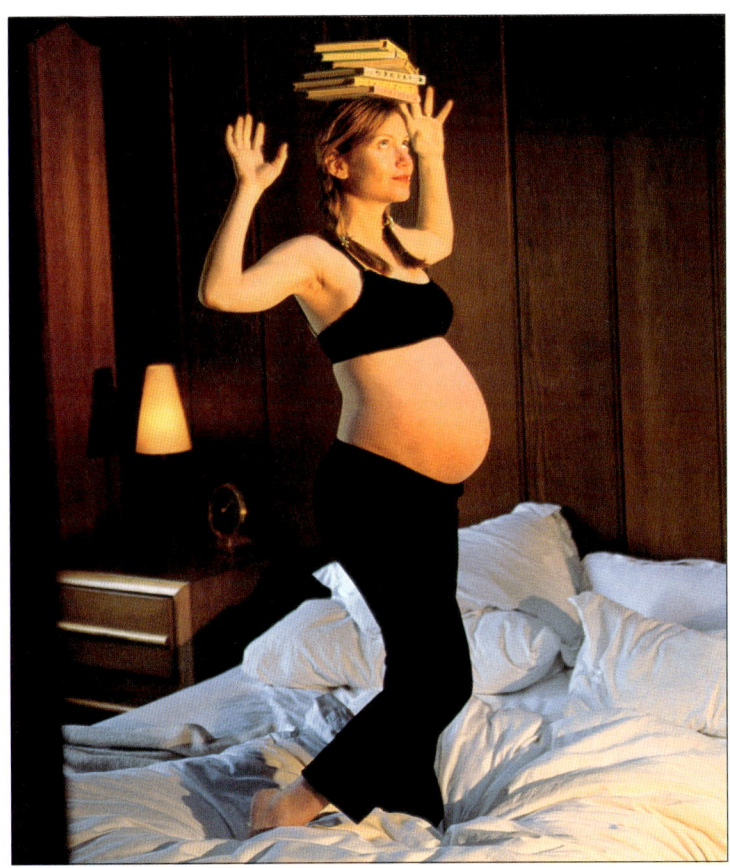

POSTURE PROBLEMS
Getting out of bed

Standing up from a lying position can be a struggle as you do not have your former flexibility. There is a method that many women find works well and protects the back.

1 Turn on to your side and swing your legs off the edge of the bed, keeping your feet together.

2 Push yourself upwards using your arms, but take care not to strain your neck. Keep your movements slow and gentle.

3 Pause for a rest while sitting on the side of the bed. When you are ready, stand normally.

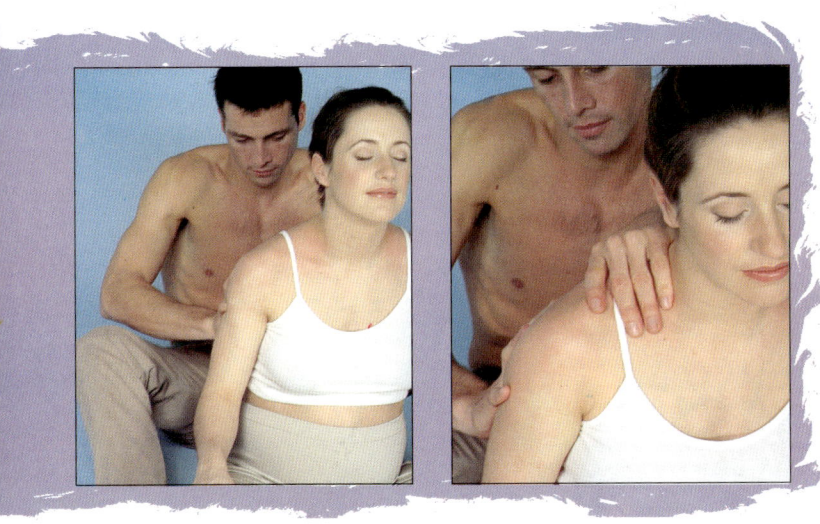

WEEK 31

Your antenatal visits will now be held every two weeks, so your midwife can carry out more frequent checks on blood pressure and urine, and monitor your baby's size and position. Don't worry if your midwife tells you the baby is still in the breech (bottom down) position. Some babies wait until as late as the 36th week to turn. If your baby continues to lie in that position, there are exercises that might help (see pages 76 and 77).

What's happening to you
• You may feel more breathless at times. This is normal – your heart and lungs have to work much harder now in providing oxygenated blood for you and your growing baby. Don't rush about or take on too much, as you'll need plenty of rest during these last two months.

Baby at 31 weeks

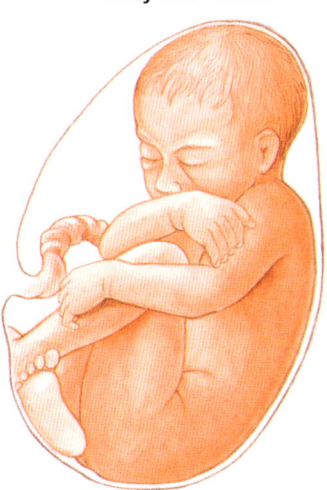

What's happening to your baby
• Your baby now weighs 1.8–2.3kg (4–5lb), and is nearly 30cm (12in) in length from head to rump.
• Many babies now lie upside down, with their heads inside the cradle of mum's pelvis, ready to be born head first.

• Your baby may already have a lot of hair on his or her head. This is especially true of dark-haired babies.

CASE NOTES

How to cope in the final weeks

Charlie is 34, and pregnant with her second child. Her first child is now three years old. She found the final stages of her pregnancy very trying.

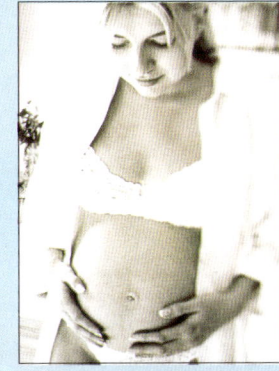

'I was utterly exhausted because I had insomnia, and would lie awake in bed all night switching positions with pillows. Then I would need a nap during the day. We hired a childminder to look after Sally for a couple of afternoons a week, and this way I could catch up on my sleep.

We had a futon in the bedroom, but we had to go out and get a proper sprung mattress and bed base because the hard futon was too uncomfortable on my hips and back. It was also far too low for me to get out of when I started to become really big. I find that having a bath in the evening is the best way of relieving the ache in my legs, and the water feels very supportive around my bump.'

Special Care

B ABIES BORN at this time have an excellent chance of survival, but they need to be constantly monitored and protected in a carefully controlled environment. The special care baby unit (SCBU) is staffed by highly specialised doctors and nurses who know how to look after newborn babies during these early, vulnerable days in the outside world.

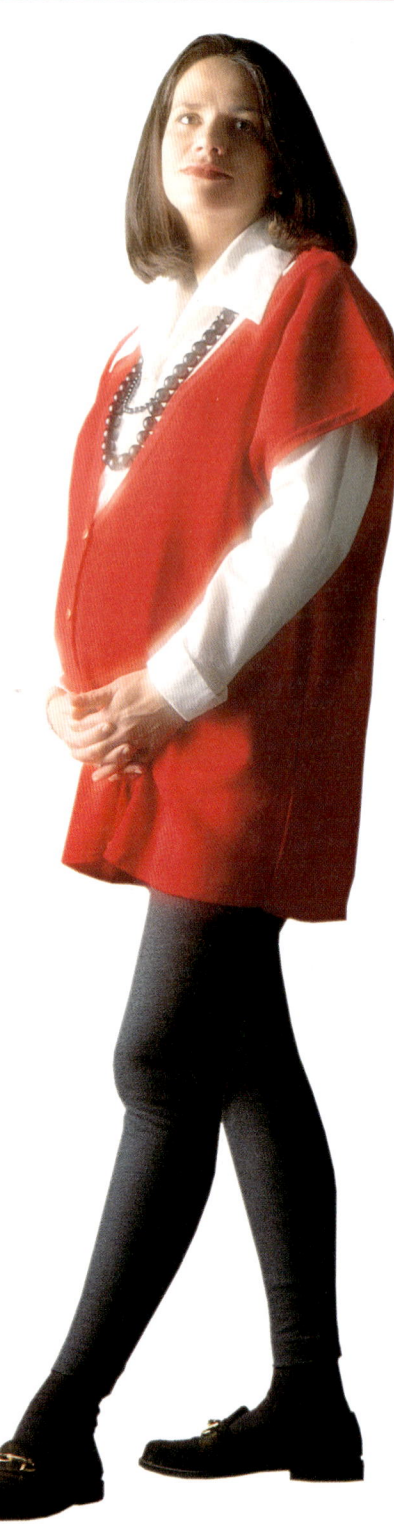

Babies who are born preterm (prematurely) or undersized may need extra care during their early weeks until they have developed sufficiently to be able to go home with their mother. Babies are generally considered to be small if they are under 2.3kg (5lb), which is the case in about 1 in 20 births, although not all such babies require special care.

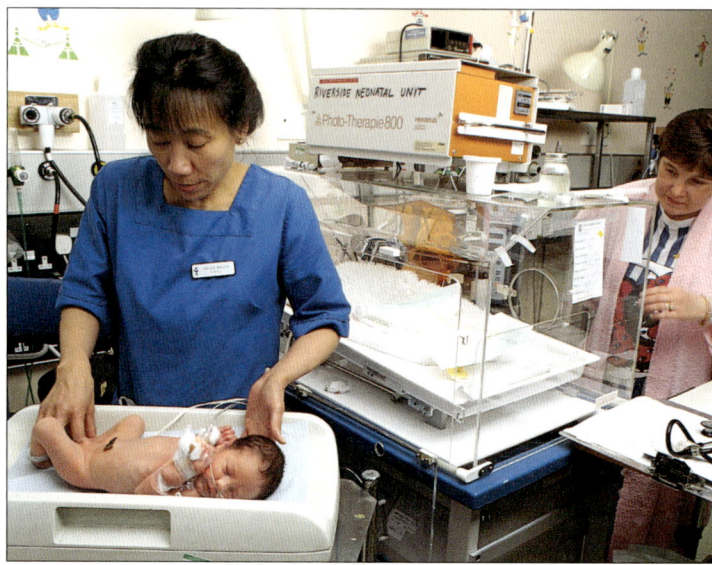

Low birth weight

There are many reasons why babies may be too small, the most common being that they have been born too early. This is often because the birth was induced at an early stage, perhaps because the health of mother or baby was at risk in some way. In other cases, premature birth may be related to abnormal hormone levels affecting the actions of the uterus. In many cases, however, the cause of premature birth is not known.

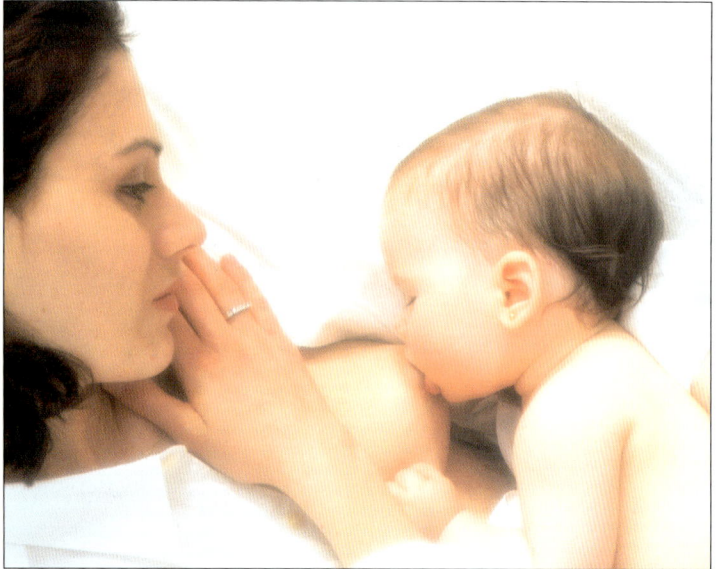

Other babies may be born small even though they have gone the full nine months. This is often the case in multiple births (see pages 50 and 51), but can also occur if the placenta was not functioning properly, or if the mother smoked, or lived a very high-stress lifestyle during her pregnancy.

Special care

If necessary, your baby will be looked after in a special care baby unit, a ward designed and staffed specifically for the care of vulnerable babies. There are particular problems relating to the care of such small and delicate babies that SCBUs are best able to deal with.

TEMPERATURE: Small or preterm babies lack sufficient body fat to regulate their body temperature efficiently and so are kept warm in an incubator until fully developed. An incubator is an enclosed cabinet, often with access holes in the side so that carers can tend to the baby's needs without having to move the infant, and mum and dad can cuddle their newborn. Special care babies are extremely vulnerable to infection, so staff and visitors must wear masks, gloves and other protective clothing at all times.

BREATHING: A baby's lungs take longer to develop in the womb than other organs, so preterm babies may have difficulty breathing. Oxygen is supplied to the baby via a small catheter (tube) inserted into the nostril. This uses controlled positive pressure to gently help the baby's lungs expand.

FEEDING: Mothers are encouraged to feed small babies breast milk as this is the ideal food, supplying all the required nutrients in the right proportions. The baby's stomach may not be able to cope with the usual feeding routine and so may be fed little and often.

A very premature or sick baby may be fed sugar water until well enough to digest milk. Sometimes the baby may be fed with a continuous drip via a small catheter, either inserted through a nostril into the stomach, or, if the digestive tract is underdeveloped, into a vein.

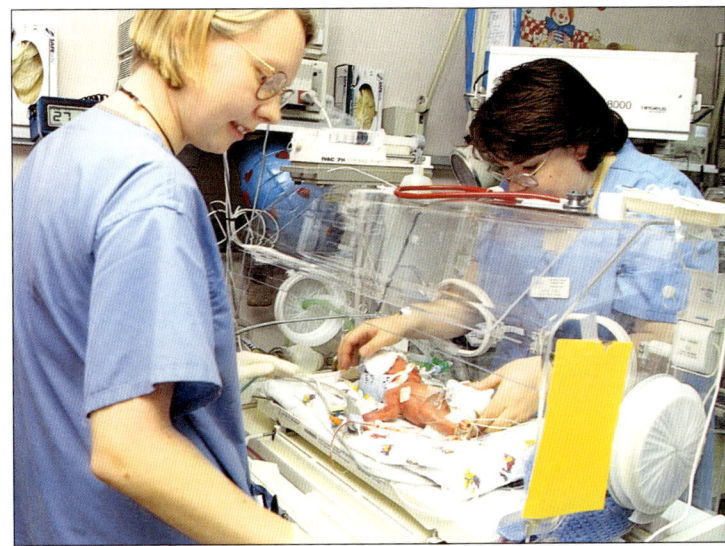

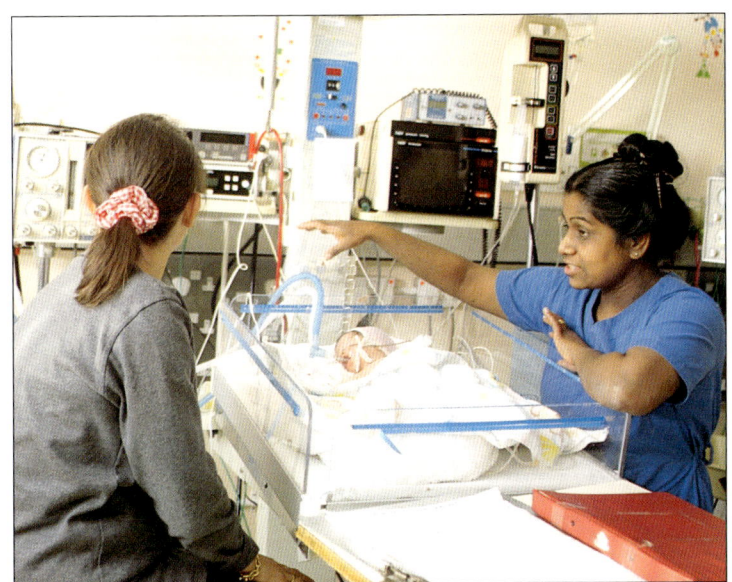

Kangaroo care – the power of a cuddle

The love and attention given to small babies by their parents is just as important as expensive hospital equipment. It has been proven that contact and reassurance, especially from the mother, is crucial if a newborn is to develop quickly. Special care baby units try to make parents feel at home so that they will spend as long as possible with their child. Mothers are encouraged to hold and feed their baby whenever possible – an approach sometimes termed 'kangaroo care' (just as kangaroos keep their babies in their pouch). Small newborns relish the chance to be near their mothers, and direct skin contact is one of the best ways to encourage bonding and development.

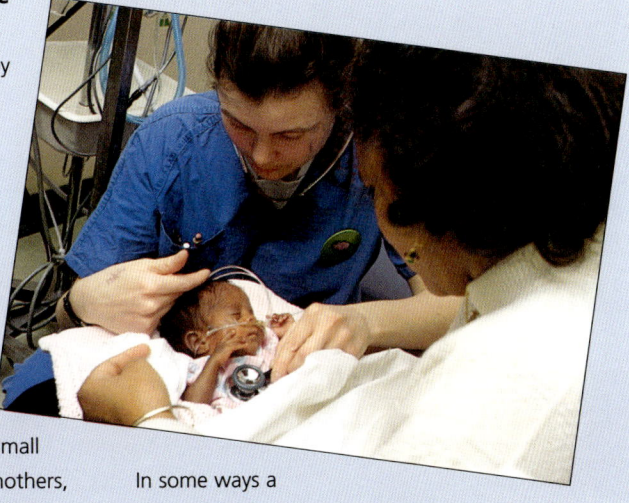

In some ways a mother's body is like an incubator, and sometimes newborns just need to be cuddled.

WEEK 32

During antenatal visits, the doctor or midwife will listen to your baby's heartbeat with a stethoscope. In the later stages of pregnancy, experienced midwives may even tell the sex of your baby by this means, because a girl's heart rate in the womb tends to be slightly faster than a boy's. An ultrasound scanner can confirm the sex of the baby, provided the operator has an unobstructed view.

What's happening to you
• You may be feeling really heavy and sluggish, and worry that your pregnancy seems never ending. In some ways, these can be the most difficult weeks as you prepare your home for the arrival of a newborn, and must wait and keep rested until you have carried your baby to term.
• You may also be feeling anxious about the birth. The best way to cope with these feelings is through action. Write a birthplan (see pages 86–91), or a letter to your unborn child explaining how you feel and what you hope for your lives together. Your partner is there to give you support, so confide in him – it is better to include him in your thoughts than shut him out. Just talking things over can make a big difference.

What's happening to your baby
• Your baby now measures 42cm (16in) and is perfectly formed.
• All the necessary layers of fat have yet to be laid down, and the lungs are still not capable of unassisted breathing.

FACT BOX
Around 6 per cent of babies weigh under 2.25kg (5lb) at birth, because they fail to develop or are premature.

DRUG RISKS

AN UNBORN baby may be affected by any substance that enters the mother's bloodstream. This is particularly so in the case of drugs, both recreational and medicinal. If, in the past, you've felt that recreational drugs or tranquillisers offer the only way to ease tension and relax, think of your unborn baby and consider other options.

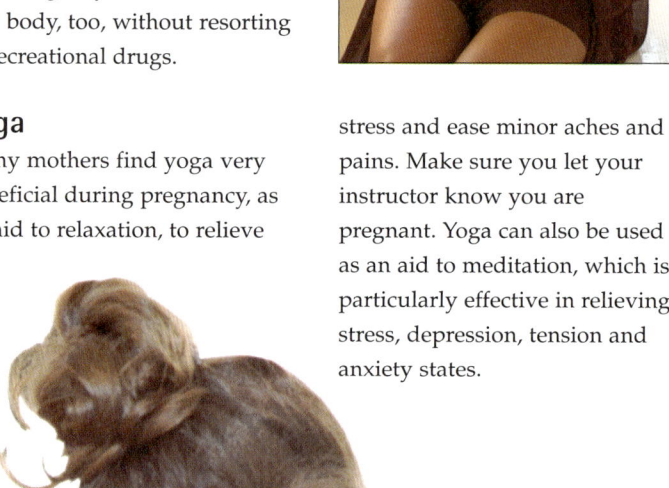

As with alcohol and smoking, recreational drugs are potentially harmful to unborn babies, whose developing bodies are particularly vulnerable to the effects of chemicals. This is a special time because the life inside you is totally dependent on you for all the care and nourishment he or she receives. This is why you have to be extra careful about what you are putting in your body.

Doctors don't always know the full effects that many drugs may have on an unborn baby, particularly those used for recreational use (such as cannabis or ecstasy). If you accept such substances into your body you may be exposing your child to unknown harms.

Safe alternatives

Even drugs that are normally considered 'safe', such as aspirin, might have an adverse effect on an unborn child. Where possible, avoid over-the-counter medications during pregnancy and try to find non-drug remedies for your symptoms. For example, you can often ease a headache by resting quietly in a darkened room, or by placing a cool moist flannel on your forehead.

A warm bath can ease back pain, and a cold compress can be used to reduce swelling and inflammation. There are many non-drug ways to relax mind and body, too, without resorting to recreational drugs.

Yoga

Many mothers find yoga very beneficial during pregnancy, as an aid to relaxation, to relieve stress and ease minor aches and pains. Make sure you let your instructor know you are pregnant. Yoga can also be used as an aid to meditation, which is particularly effective in relieving stress, depression, tension and anxiety states.

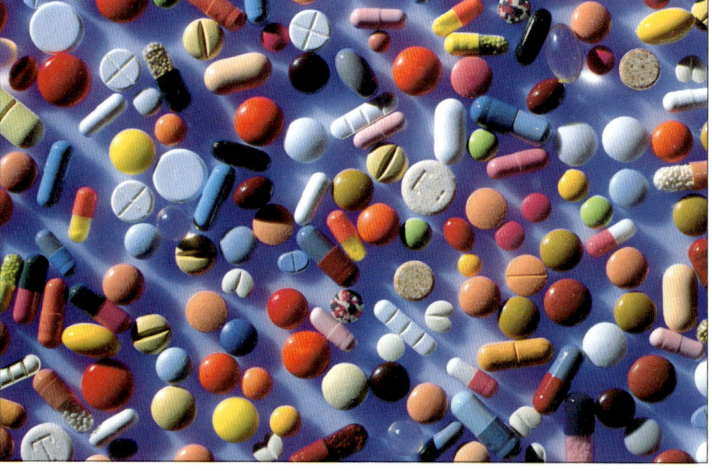

It is best to avoid drugs during pregnancy if you can, unless you really must take medication for a chronic condition such as diabetes or epilepsy.

Drug chart

Avoid drugs in pregnancy if possible and always seek your doctor's advice before taking any drug. Never stop taking a prescription medicine without first consulting your doctor, however, as you or your baby may be harmed if some disorders, such as asthma or diabetes, are not properly controlled.

Drug	Uses	Comments
Amphetamines	*Stimulant*	Can cause fetal defects.
Anabolic steroids	*Body building*	Gives female fetus masculine characteristics.
Antihistamines	*Vomiting/allergies*	Use only those types recommended for pregnant women.
Aspirin	*Painkiller/eases inflammation*	Avoid in third trimester, if possible, as high doses may affect labour and fetus.
Cannabis	*Recreation*	Risk of chromosomal and brain damage to fetus. Often used with tobacco which can cause low birth weight babies.
Cocaine	*Stimulant*	Leads to underweight, addicted babies.
Codeine	*Painkiller*	Avoid in third trimester, if possible, as it can adversely affect mother in labour and a newborn baby's breathing.
Diuretics	*Diet pills/high blood pressure*	Can cause fetal blood problems and other disorders. (Not prescribed in pregnancy.)
Ibuprofen	*Painkiller/eases inflammation*	Avoid in third trimester, if possible, as high doses may affect labour and fetus.
LSD	*Hallucinogenic*	Causes miscarriage/premature labour.
Paracetamol	*Painkiller/reduces fever*	Not known to be harmful but avoid prolonged or excessive use.
Sleeping pills	*Induce sleep*	Avoid, especially in the first and third trimesters, or use only on doctor's advice.
Tranquillisers	*Anti-stress/anxiety*	Avoid if possible, especially in third trimester. Otherwise, use only on doctor's advice as may cause breathing and other difficulties in newborns.

Floatation Tank

Also known as a floatarium, this involves floating in a sound-proof, light-proof tank. Many women find that it aids stress relief and peace of mind as they lie there peacefully, shut off from telephones, traffic and the other noisy trappings of the modern world.

Aromatherapy

Many of the oils used in aromatherapy have relaxing and calming properties and can ease tension headaches, especially when used in a soothing massage. Some oils may have harmful effects in pregnancy, however, so always go to a qualified aromatherapist and be sure to say that you are pregnant.

You may be able to distinguish the different parts of your baby's body, such as the head, rump, elbow or foot, without your midwife's help. Your baby's prods are much stronger, and may cause a sharp intake of breath. You may need to sit for a while if your baby is feeling really energetic and giving you a firm kicking.

What's happening to you
• Your lower ribs or pelvis may be feeling particularly sore at the moment, in which case hot water bottles (not too hot) or a warm bath may help.

What's happening to your baby
• Your baby is now too big to move around much in your womb.
• Your baby's position (most likely head down) will probably be the one he or she adopts for birth.
• Your baby may go through periods of jerking around repeatedly, often due to hiccups. This can occur to unborn babies if they gulp a little too much of the amniotic fluid as they practise their swallowing reflex.
• Your baby weighs 2kg (4½)lb and is about 32cm (12in) long from the top of the head to the rump.

HOME SAFETY

BABIES DEVELOP very quickly. By the time your child is six months old, he or she will be crawling and exploring your home, and will be very curious about this new world. Now is a good time to look at your home from your child's perspective and take steps to eliminate any potential dangers you may find.

Accident statistics show that children are most at risk between the ages of 12 and 24 months. At this age they are mobile, active and curious, but do not yet understand the hidden dangers lurking inside every home. As parents, you'll naturally try to ensure that your child is well supervised – but you can't keep a child under surveillance all the time. For your child's safety – and your own peace of mind – think about the steps you can take to make your home a 'baby-friendly' zone.

Basic safety

Try this experiment: crawl around your home and imagine how a baby will see it. Anything small and unusual will probably be placed inside the child's mouth, any dangling wires will be grabbed, any handles, drawers or cupboard doors will be pulled open to reveal what is inside. Children's minds are like a sponge – soaking up information about the world around them. They are insatiably curious, and you cannot control this impulse. There are certain minimum steps you should take, and once you start to think about home safety you'll probably come up with lots more.

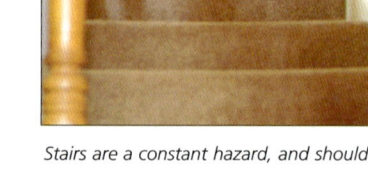

Stairs are a constant hazard, and should always be blocked off with a stairgate, even if your baby can only crawl.

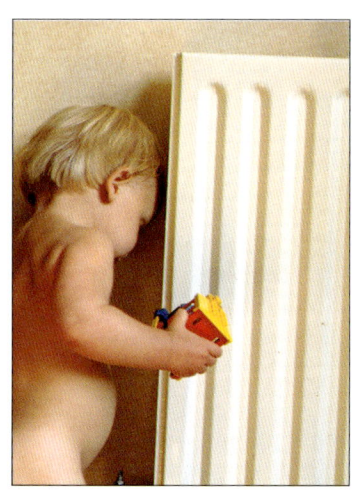

Radiators can be very dangerous to a baby's thinner and more delicate skin.

Blades

All sharp-edged items such as razor blades, tools and kitchen utensils should be stored out of reach, up high on hooks or in a cabinet, or in a childproof drawer or locked tool box.

Doors

Fit door jammers to prevent the child's fingers getting trapped if the door suddenly blows shut.

Electric sockets

Fit a socket guard to any electric outlet that a child can reach and switch off when not in use.

Fires and heaters

Open fires should have a guard that covers the whole hearth –

babies can burn their fingers on any hot surface. Electric and portable gas heaters should be firmly secured as well as covered by a guard. Make sure radiators are not too hot or cover them with a guard.

Fire safety

Fit smoke detectors throughout the home, checking periodically that the batteries work.

Locks

All doors and drawers up to 1m (around 3ft) above the floor should be fitted with childproof locks. Fit them now so that all the adults in the house can get used to them.

Overheating

Don't use a duvet or thick woollen blanket in the cot or crib until the baby is at least one

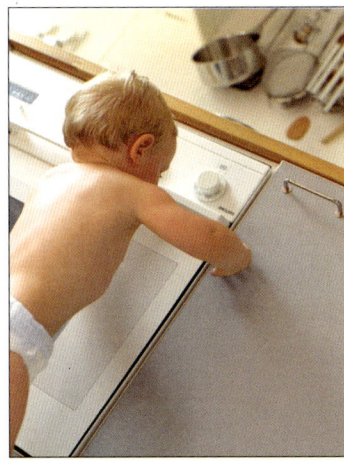

year old, as overheating is thought by some experts to be an important factor in cot death.

Poisons

All potentially toxic substances should be kept out of reach or locked up. This not only includes hazardous chemicals such as bleach, toilet cleaner and pesticide – contraceptive

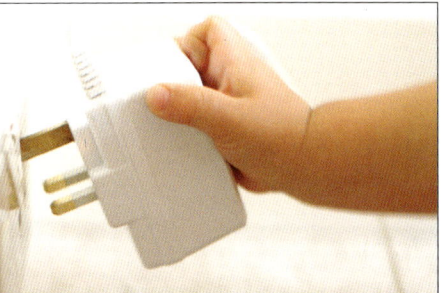

Fitting plug covers is a cheap and effective idea, as are cupboard guards. You should never leave your child playing unattended.

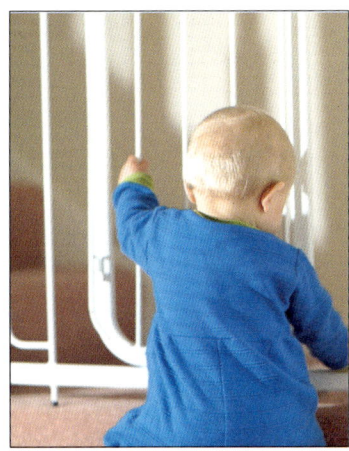

pills and even vitamin pills can be hazardous to a child. Objects small enough to be swallowed – less than 2–3cm (1in) wide – such as coins and marbles, should also be kept out of reach.

Scalding

A baby's skin is very vulnerable to burns – even a cup of tea can scald. Get into the habit of placing hot drinks and boiling kettles out of reach. Always turn saucepan handles away from the cooker edge or fit a pan guard. Check that the hot water thermostat is not set too high.

Smoking

Don't allow smoking in the nursery, and preferably not in the house.

Stairs

Even short flights of stairs and steps should be protected by safety gates – at the top and bottom. Fit them now so you can practise using them before the baby arrives.

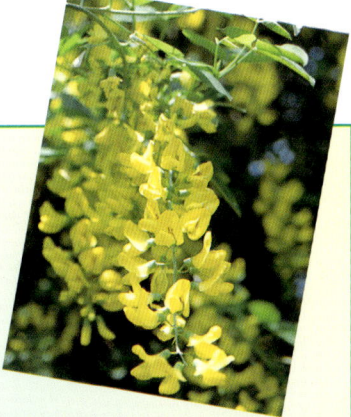

Plant safety – poisonous flora

Many house and garden plants are harmful to infants if eaten or, in some cases, touched. Symptoms and signs include burns and swelling to the skin, mouth and throat, abdominal pain, and diarrhoea. If you suspect your child may have been affected, seek emergency medical aid immediately and take a piece of the plant with you so it can be identified. Check that houseplants and garden plants are safe or remove them if in any doubt.

Toxic houseplants include: dumb cane (*Dieffenbachia*), hyacinth (*Hyathincus*), ivy (*Hedera*), poinsettia (*Euphorbia pulcherrima*), rubber plant (*Ficus*), Swiss cheese plant (*Monstera*) and wandering Jew (*Tradescantia*).

Toxic garden plants include: bluebell (*Endymion*), cotoneaster, delphinium, euphorbia, laburnum (pictured above right), lupin (*Lupinus*), morning glory (*Ipomoea*), snowdrop (*Galanthus*), and wisteria.

WEEK 34

Your baby's head may have engaged into your pelvis by now – the head nestles like an egg in an eggcup. If your baby bumps your pelvic bone, or if you sit down suddenly, you may experience what feel like little shocks in your groin, or a buzzing sensation in your vagina.

What's happening to you
• Once your baby's head engages, you'll find breathing easier as there is more room above your abdomen for your diaphragm and internal organs.
• You may also find that if you have been suffering from heartburn this will ease up.
• Your visits to the lavatory will be as frequent as ever – there is now little space for your bladder, which has to be emptied much more frequently.

What's happening to your baby
• Your baby will be kicking less, as he or she cannot move around as freely as a month ago. Instead, your baby will shuffle and 'squirm', which is the most he or she can do curled tightly inside you with the legs tucked tightly underneath the body.
• The baby's face and body has a smoother and more rounded appearance now because of the thicker layer of fat under the skin.

Mother and uterus at 34 weeks

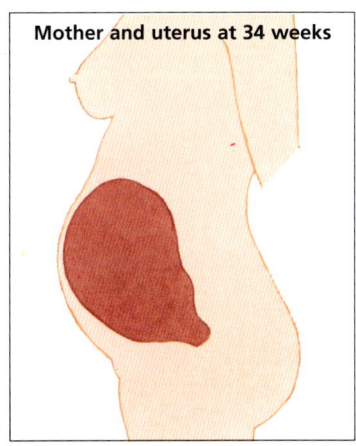

FETAL POSITIONING

NOW IS A good time to start preparing mentally and physically for the delivery. There are steps you can take to help delivery go as smoothly as possible, such as trying to ensure that your baby is in the right position prior to birth. This can be helped by doing some simple exercises.

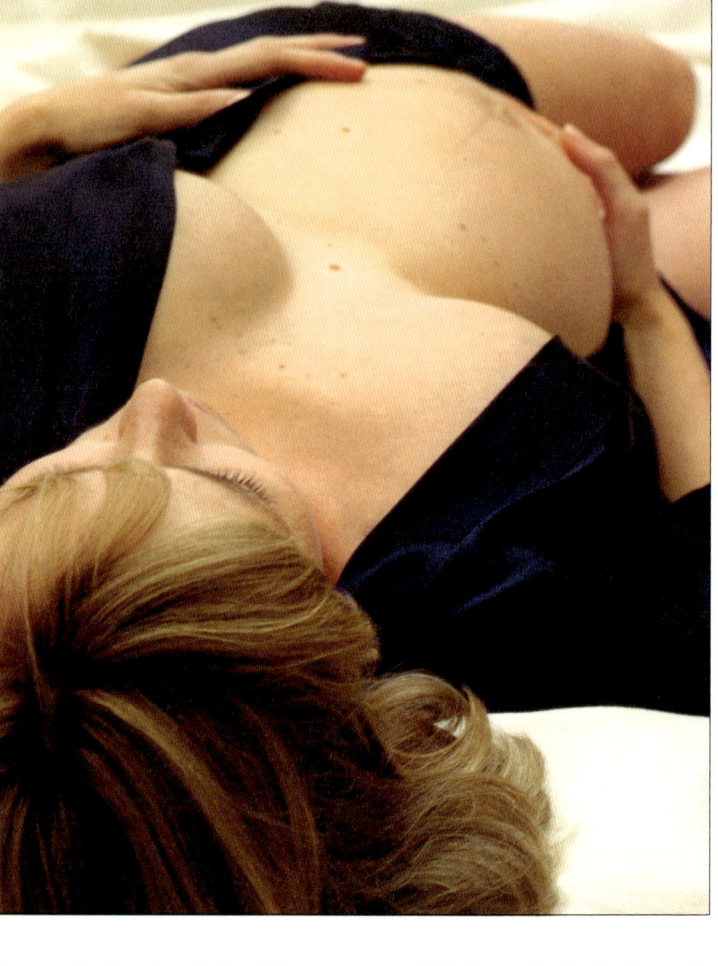

It is likely that within the next two weeks (if not already) your baby will have turned into the head-down position, ready for birth. Only around 5 per cent of babies are still in the breech (bottom down) position by 37 weeks. Some babies turn just before their birth (to keep mum guessing!).

Delivery decisions

If your baby is still in the breech position by the estimated date, the chances are that delivery will be by Caesarean section. It is possible to deliver breech babies vaginally, which many mums find satisfying and a real achievement. The midwife's main concern, however, is that this is a much more difficult delivery, and increases the risk to the baby who may, for example, be deprived of oxygen during the birth.

The size of the mother's pelvis is taken into account when considering the safest kind of delivery she can be expected to undergo. As a general rule, the wider the better – hence the expression 'child-bearing hips'.

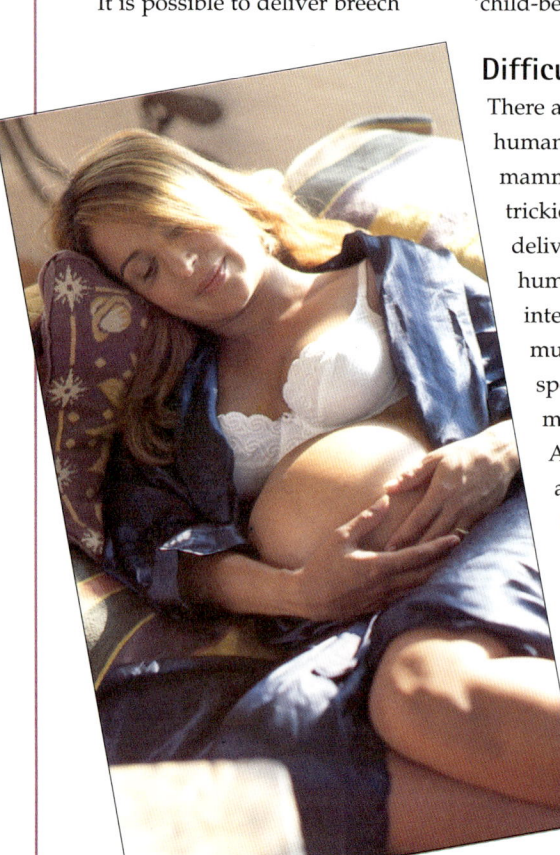

Difficult passage

There are several reasons why humans, compared with other mammals, can experience trickier and longer deliveries. For one reason, human babies are highly intelligent, so the head is much bigger, relatively speaking, than other mammal offspring.

Another reason is that, as upright walkers, the human pelvis tips forward. As a result, during the birth a baby has to negotiate a less direct route – a sort of S-bend – to the outside world. The baby does this by making a half-turn as the head and shoulders emerge. People today also spend less time walking than previous generations (thanks to cars), so babies are less likely to 'drop' into the right place.

Turning baby

There are many ways you can encourage your baby to be in the right place at the right time:

WALKING: This not only helps mums to keep fit but is also comforting for babies who like the rocking motion it produces. Walking may also encourage a baby to turn, if still in the breech position, and the head to engage in the pelvis. The head is the heaviest part of his body and so will naturally tend to gravitate towards the bottom of the uterus. (Swimming the breaststroke can also encourage this to occur.)

ANTENATAL CLASSES: Exercises to help position the baby prior to birth are taught at antenatal classes. You will also learn breathing and relaxation techniques that are designed to help you get through labour. These techniques are of great benefit in aiding the delivery and will also help take your mind off the contractions (see pages 86–91).

YOGA: Many yoga classes for pregnant women include positions specifically designed to help the baby drop into the right position. These include being on all fours, or sitting so that the pelvis is tilted forward.

AT HOME: If your baby is still in the breech position, there are other steps you can take each day that may be effective:
• Crawl on your hands and knees for up to 10 minutes.
• Sleep on your left side.
• Use beanbags to lean into, to help your pelvis tip forward.
• Sit with your knees lower than your hips.

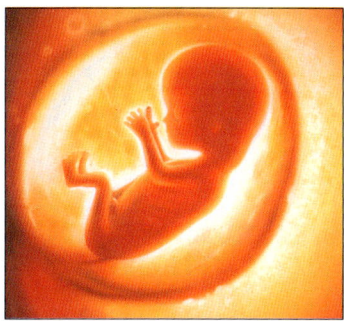

You can see from the comparison of fetuses at 16 weeks (above) and at 35 weeks (see panel below) how much less room there is for your baby to move around inside the womb.

Ideal position?

Occipito anterior is the term used to describe the baby's ideal position for delivery – head down, engaged into the pelvis, with the baby's back on the left side of the mother's abdomen, and the back of the head against the front of the mother's pelvis.

FACT BOX

Around 15 per cent of babies are still in the breech position by week 32. Of these, most (70 per cent) turn before it is time to be born.

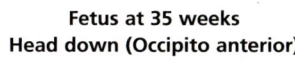

**Fetus at 35 weeks
Head down (Occipito anterior)**

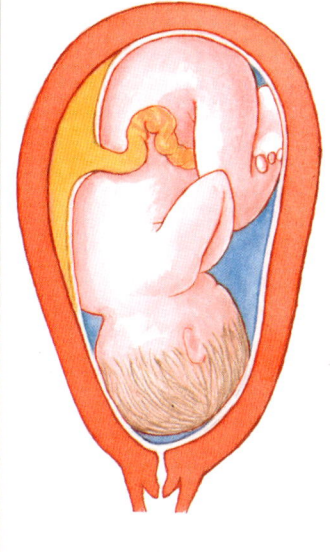

**Fetus at 35 weeks
Breech**

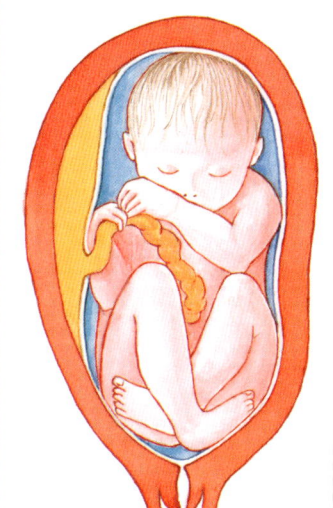

WEEK 35

Every day counts to give your baby the best possible start in life. Although fully developed by now, your baby needs these extra few weeks to gather strength for the birth and life in the outside world (although most babies born after 35 weeks have a very good chance of doing fine).

What's happening to you
• Your pelvic joints are softening in preparation for the birth so that your body copes better with the delivery.
• By now, your blood volume has increased by up to 40 per cent to cope with the extra needs of your changing body as well as the extra needs of your growing baby, which can sometimes make you feel breathless.
• You may find it harder to sleep, and sometimes feel restless. However, try to get as much rest as possible in the final weeks.

What's happening to your baby
• Your baby now weighs 2.2–2.5kg (5–5½lb) and is 34cm (13½in) from crown to rump.
• To your baby, sunlight appears as a red glow.
• Your baby is receiving antibodies from your system via the placenta. This gives some measure of protection against infection after the birth. If you breastfeed, your baby continues to receive antibodies through your breast milk, which can help to continue the protection for up to six weeks. Breast milk is beneficial in many other ways, too, so you should try to continue to feed your baby yourself for as long as possible.

THE NAMING GAME

WHAT'S IN a name? Well, the name parents give their children may stay with them for the rest of their lives. The name also has implications for the child-parent relationship: in some ways they come to regard their name as their parent's 'opinion' of them. It is worth giving some serious thought to this tricky issue.

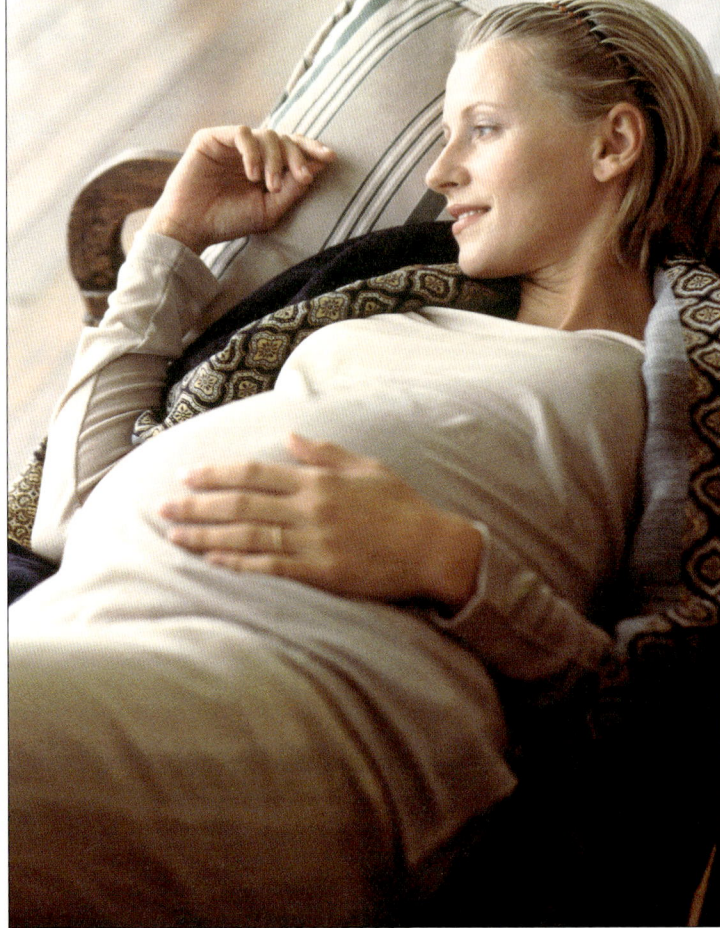

When choosing your baby's name there are many pitfalls to be wary of which, if you are not careful, can lead to later embarrassment and confusion. Before committing your baby's name to the birth certificate, try to look at all the implications of your choice.

Naming tips

You do not have to stick to just one 'given' name – second, third, or more names can be useful. They give the child a more original identity, so helping to avoid confusion, they provide a way of paying tribute to a relative or friend, and they offer children other choices if they don't like the first name they have been given.

EASE OF USE: The name should be relatively easy to spell and pronounce if you want your child to master it quickly and

not be forever spelling it out to uncomprehending strangers.

DIMINUTIVES: Whether you wish it or not, first names often get shortened, as a sign of friendship, to show familiarity – or to make fun. When thinking about a name, consider whether it has a diminutive that you would be happy with if it became the norm for your child. Alternatively, you could choose a name that is too short to be shortened further.

INITIALS: Check whether the initials of first, middle and surname spell out an embarrassing word, or have any other unfortunate connotation.

CELEBRITY NAMES: If you are considering naming your baby after a favourite celebrity, try to choose one that will not seem dated over time and make your child the butt of jokes at school.

UNISEX: Some popular names, such as Ashley, Chris, Francis (Frances), Jan, Kim, and Lesley (Leslie), can be used both for boys and girls. A unisex name might seem useful if

you don't yet know the sex of your child, but bear in mind it may lead to confusion in later life and can be embarrassing.

Popular western names

There is now greater similarity in the list of most popular names among the English-speaking countries, possibly because of the effect of an increasingly global media.

On the next page we show the top 50 boys names and top 50 girls names recorded in UK register offices, but you will find that many are also popular as far apart as North America, and Australasia. Some are relative newcomers, but most have been popular for many years.

WEEK 36

The top 100 names in the UK

Girls' names

Abigail	Chelsea	Georgia	Lauren	Paige
Alexandra	Chloe	Georgina	Leah	Phoebe
Alice	Courteney	Grace	Louise	Rachel
Amber	Danielle	Hannah	Lucy	Rebecca
Amelia	Eleanor	Holly	Lydia	Samantha
Amy	Elizabeth	Jade	Megan	Sarah
Anna	Ella	Jasmine	Molly	Shannon
Bethany	Ellie	Jessica	Natasha	Sophie
Caitlin	Emily	Katie	Nicole	Victoria
Charlotte	Emma	Laura	Olivia	Zoe

Boys' names

Aaron	Cameron	George	Joshua	Nathan
Adam	Charles	Harry	Kieran	Oliver
Alex	Charlie	Jack	Kyle	Owen
Alexander	Christopher	Jacob	Lewis	Reece
Andrew	Connor	Jake	Liam	Robert
Ben	Daniel	James	Luke	Ryan
Benjamin	David	Jamie	Matthew	Sam
Bradley	Dylan	Jonathan	Max	Samuel
Brandon	Edward	Jordan	Michael	Thomas
Callum	Ethan	Joseph	Mohammed	William

You will be seeing your midwife or specialist once a week now as you approach the final phase of your pregnancy. This may be a troublesome time for you: you've been quite heavy for a while now, and may be slightly anxious about the birth ahead, and wondering how you will care for a newborn baby 24 hours a day. Your partner should try to relax and reassure you and help you as much as possible so you can concentrate on preparing for the birth.

What's happening to you

• You may find that you are clumsier than usual, and feeling quite off-balance. This is normal – your bump is now so big that you have to lean back to offset the weight of the baby. Tying shoes may be a real problem, so get someone to help you or wear slip-ons for the last few weeks.

FACT BOX Around 90 per cent of Western children are named from the same limited pool year after year.

What's happening to your baby

• Your baby is 45cm (18in) long and weighs nearly 2.7kg (6lb).

• The baby's intestines are filled with a dark substance called meconium, which is made up of secretions from the baby's glands, and cells discarded as the body develops. The baby voids this substance during or straight after the birth. It is possible for babies to inhale meconium as they are being born, which may result in a lung infection. Midwives watch out for this problem and may use a special tube after birth to suck out any material that has entered the baby's airway.

World names and international traditions

Muslim names are generally descriptive, and may be linked to religious themes. For example, Salim means safe, Bakr means young camel, Fatima means the prophet's favourite daughter. Mohammed (the Prophet) is often used as an act of devotion, as is Abd-Allah (servant of Allah), and Ahmad (to praise Allah).

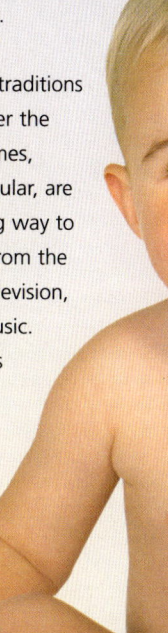

Hindu and Sikh names can also have many religious connections. For example, the girl's name Gita means 'singing praises'.

Catholic culture tends to feature saints names prominently, such as Sebastian, Patrick and David for boys. Mary, the most common girl's name, was once attached as a standard prefix (such as Mary-Ben) in some Catholic cultures.

Chinese make the first name the family title and the second is a name shared by all relatives of a particular generation. The third name is

individual to each child and tends to be descriptive: Chiang (boy, strong), Shu (girl, good) and Ying (girl, flower).

Western naming traditions have changed over the years. Biblical names, although still popular, are increasingly giving way to celebrity names from the worlds of film, television, sport and pop music. Descriptive names such as Sky, Rainbow and River have also risen in popularity since the 1960s.

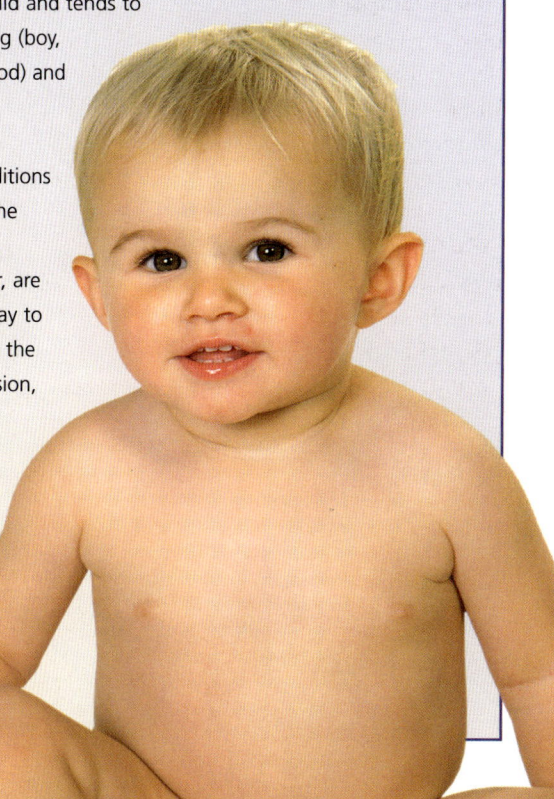

PREGNANCY FAQS

THE PROCESS of pregnancy and childbirth can seem extremely complicated, with high-tech screening and monitoring equipment, rigorous laboratory tests, and confusing terminology. The doctor and midwife will be happy to answer any queries you may have, but it may also help you to know what are some of the most frequently asked questions (FAQs).

FACT BOX

Even if your baby is delivered by Caesarean section on this occasion, it does not automatically rule out having a future baby by vaginal birth.

Why is my blood pressure checked?

High blood pressure can cause complications and may need to be treated with medication. High blood pressure is also a possible indicator of pre-eclampsia, along with oedema (fluid retention in the tissues), and protein in the urine. Pre-eclampsia affects 1 in 20 women, usually in the second half of the pregnancy. In most cases it is mild but the mother will need to be closely monitored and may be advised to rest in bed.

Severe pre-eclampsia is potentially very harmful to mother and baby and can lead to eclampsia, in which the woman suffers seizures and may lapse into coma.

Regular monitoring of pregnant women has greatly reduced the risk of pre-eclampsia developing to this serious stage.

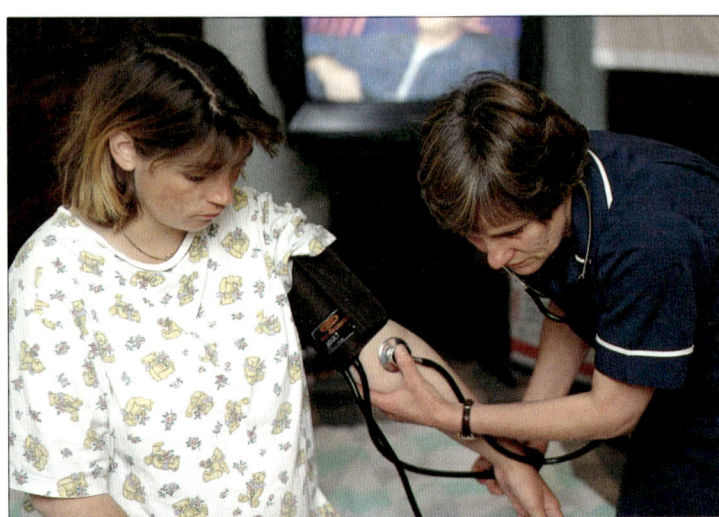

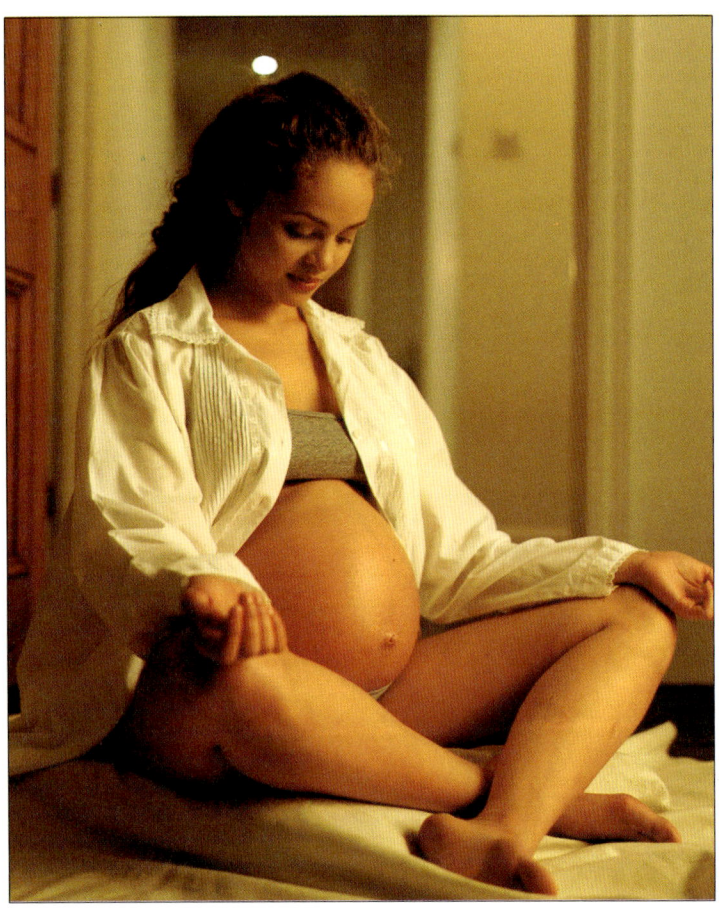

Does sugar in my urine mean I am diabetic?

Sugar in the urine can indicate diabetes but is not in itself conclusive. Some pregnant women have kidneys which are more likely to temporarily 'leak' than normal, and the result is that excess sugar is excreted in their urine. If sugar repeatedly shows up in urine samples, which are taken at antenatal visits, then you may undergo other tests.

It is quite common for mild diabetes to develop in the second half of pregnancy (called gestational diabetes) and for blood sugar levels to return to pre-pregnancy levels after the birth. Women with diabetes must be closely monitored during pregnancy and may need medication if they develop signs that their insulin levels are not sufficient.

Why does the midwife feel my bump?

Midwives do this to assess the growth of the baby, and the position in which he or she is lying. Experienced midwives can tell a lot from gently feeling around your abdomen. They can compare the size of your uterus with your expected delivery date to check how the baby is progressing.

After 28–30 weeks, they will be monitoring the position of the baby, as breech or transverse (lying across the womb) positions make the delivery more complicated unless the baby can be turned round in time.

How do I know if my symptoms are normal?

Pregnancy can be a trying time for mums-to-be and you can expect to experience any of a number of symptoms including

SEEING THE DOCTOR
How to prepare

It's your pregnancy, so don't be afraid to ask the doctor questions. It's easy to forget to ask something important – particularly if you're a first-time mother and feeling nervous – so write down a list of questions before your appointment. Apart from the obvious 'Is everything all right with my pregnancy?' consider the following points.

- What tests will I need?
- Are there any special measures I need to take?
- What forms of pain relief can I have in labour?
- Can my partner stay with me?
- What are the chances that I'll need a Caesarean section operation?
- How long will I be in hospital afterwards?

Of course, this list is not exhaustive. Depending on your particular circumstances you may have other questions you want to ask.

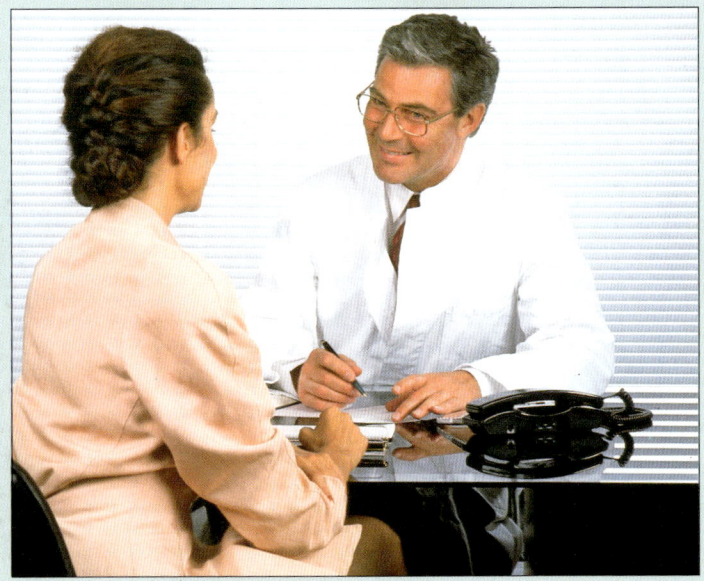

You will now be thinking about your delivery and planning for the imminent addition to your family. If you are having your baby in hospital it is a good idea to have your bag packed now so you are ready. Getting prepared can help you to feel more relaxed and settled in your mind about what lies ahead.

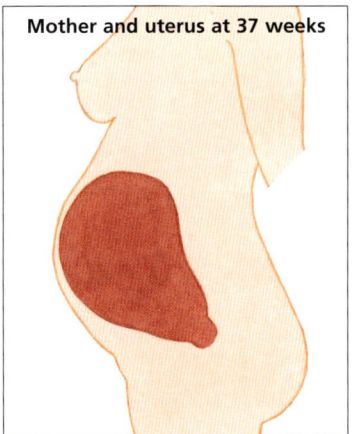

Mother and uterus at 37 weeks

What's happening to you
- It is quite normal to find yourself cleaning out a cupboard or dusting everything in the house. This is called the 'nesting instinct' because it is akin to birds preparing their nest for the arrival of eggs. Take care not to overdo it, though.

What's happening to your baby
- Your baby's last few weeks in the womb are spent putting on weight at a rapid rate – up to 28g (1oz) per day. No wonder you're feeling hungry!
- Your baby has to curl up tighter and tighter inside you in order to make use of every last bit of available space.

fatigue, nausea, headache, aching and swelling. Usually these problems are relatively mild and pass quickly.

Nevertheless, it is a good idea to make a note of any symptoms and tell your doctor or midwife at your next scheduled visit. They have the experience to judge how serious these symptoms may be. Of more concern are symptoms that are very severe or develop rapidly.

Contact your doctor promptly if you experience any of the following: blurred vision; severe persistent headache or abdominal pain; a temperature of over 37.8 °C (100 °F); sudden swelling of the face, hands, legs or feet; severe or repeated vomiting; inability to urinate; or bleeding or fluid loss from the vagina.

Is a 'low-lying placenta' a problem?

During your first ultrasound scan, the operator or your doctor may refer to your placenta as 'low-lying'. In some cases this may lead to complications. For example, the placenta may become detached from the uterine wall, causing bleeding, or it can cover the cervix and block the baby's exit from the uterus.

If a vaginal birth does not seem possible, a Caesarean section will be performed. However, most 'low-lying' placentas do not cause problems.

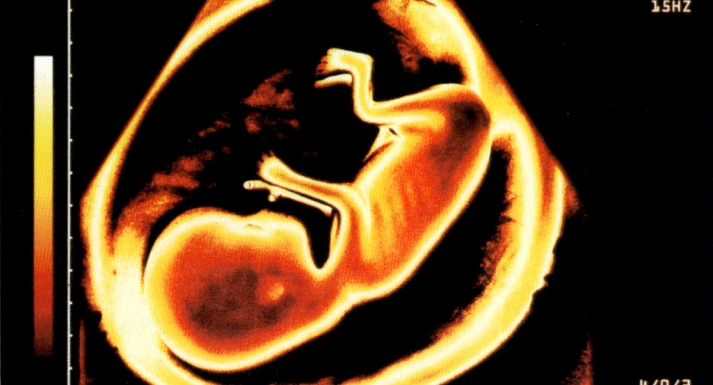

If you have a low-lying placenta, ultrasound will usually identify it.

FACT BOX
Your baby has been perfectly formed for a while – the last weeks are just spent increasing in weight and strength.

DELIVERY ROOM

YOU'LL SHORTLY be offered a tour of the delivery room as part of the maternity hospital's antenatal programme. This is an ideal time to familiarise yourself with the equipment and layout of the room, so they won't seem so intimidating when you return to have your baby – remember, you may not have time to ask questions during the delivery.

In many hospitals, labour and delivery take place in the same room. However, procedures can vary and it may be that when you are admitted to hospital, you'll go to an antenatal ward for the first stage, and then to the delivery room once the second stage of labour has started, and remain there until after the birth. You will then be taken to the postnatal ward.

The equipment

The delivery room can seem rather daunting when you see it for the first time, even though hospitals now make an effort to appear less remote and intimidating by using pictures, homely décor and furnishings, and soft lighting. Although hospital procedures can vary a little, the equipment used is very similar.

The bed

This is specially designed to give women a choice of birth position. It will usually divide in the middle to allow you to sit up during delivery, or to lie on your back with your feet in stirrups. As an alternative, some hospitals provide a birth chair. This can be tipped back and has an open-hole seat through which the baby can be delivered.

The delivery trolley

This contains the delivery equipment for your midwife and doctor. The trolley also holds forceps and vacuum extraction (Ventouse) equipment to assist delivery; a clip to seal the baby's umbilical cord after it is cut; a receptacle for the placenta, which is examined by the midwife to make sure it is complete.

Monitors

There will be an external monitor, attached to a band that goes round the mother's abdomen, which measures the frequency and strength of contractions. There is also an internal fetal monitor – a small electrode that attaches to the baby's head as he or she passes down the birth canal. This records the strength and speed of the baby's heartbeat.

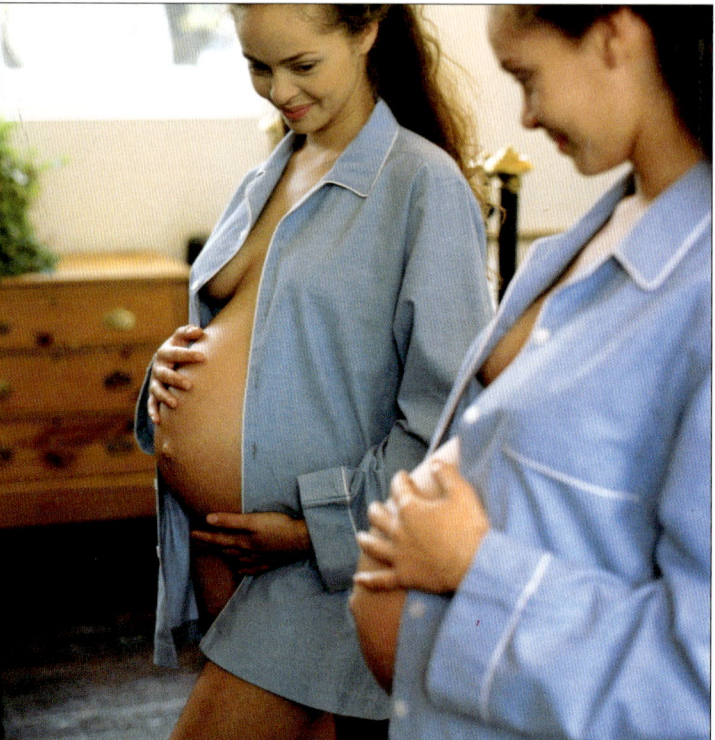

A typical delivery room in a hospital.

Entonox

A mask, attached by tube to the wall, allows you to take in pain-relieving Entonox (a mixture of nitrous oxide and oxygen) during labour and delivery. You'll normally be allowed to decide for yourself how much to take.

Clock and scales

The clock is used to record the time of birth and to time the baby's breaths per minute, and the scales measure the baby's weight.

Resuscitation trolley

Once the baby is born, the midwife will place him or her on the resuscitation trolley to assess the infant's health and wellbeing. This assessment includes the Apgar score – a measure of how responsive the baby is after the birth. This trolley also includes equipment to help clear the baby's airway and to assist breathing, if necessary.

The basinet

This is a special baby trolley that is used to carry your newborn to the postnatal ward with you. It will include a card to identify the baby and include details such as the first names (if chosen), surname, date of birth, birth weight and length. As an extra safeguard, your baby will also have wrist and ankle tags with identification details.

Birth journey

For the coming journey from the womb down the birth canal to be born, your baby's head will nestle inside your pelvis. This is called 'engaging'. You will feel that it is suddenly easier to breathe when this happens. Your baby's head is properly engaged when it sits inside the pelvic ring, rather than resting above it.

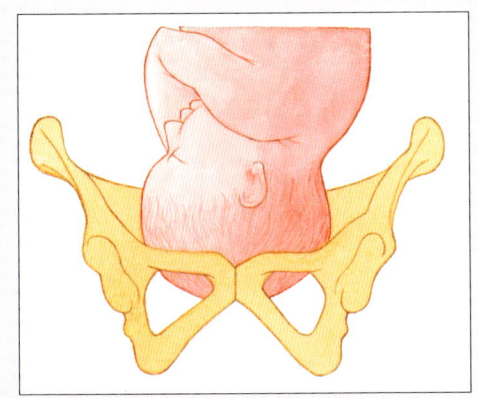

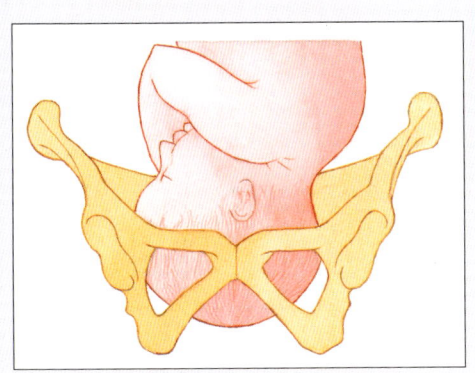

BIRTH VENUE
Home or hospital?

Unless there are special circumstances in your case, there is no reason why you shouldn't give birth at home, if you choose. Home births can be organised via your midwife, but this should be done well in advance of your due date. Some women prefer this option because they believe that home births create a more relaxed atmosphere where the mother can feel in control of events. However, it is more usual for first deliveries to take place in hospital.

The advantage of a hospital delivery is that midwives and doctors are always on hand should any emergency arise, which can be a great comfort to you and your partner. Also, there is a wider range of pain relief options available, such as an epidural (see pages 90 and 91), than could be provided at home.

Take the opportunity to visit your local maternity ward. Familiarising yourself with a delivery suite will really help to prepare you for the big day.

WEEK 38

You will now be thinking about the kind of labour and delivery you want (see pages 86–91). It is a good idea to write a birthplan at this stage so you have plenty of time to think through your options. This is also the best way of letting your partner, midwife and doctor know your preferences so that they have plenty of time to make all necessary arrangements.

What's happening to you
• You may feel rather heavy and sluggish at times, and may be worried that you won't have enough energy for the delivery. Don't worry, the mother's body always rises to the occasion and ensures you have plenty of strength. This 'winding down' prior to delivery is a way of conserving energy.
• The Braxton Hicks' contractions are much stronger and more rapid now as your body prepares for labour.
• There is over 1 litre (1¾pt) of amniotic fluid in your uterus.
• The placenta has grown to around 25cm (10in) in diameter and about 3cm (just over 1in) thick. It will soon start to shrink in preparation for the birth.

What's happening to your baby
• Your baby is plump, even chubby, as he or she has been gaining weight very rapidly over the last few weeks.
• The skin on your baby's hands and feet is wrinkled after nine months in amniotic fluid.

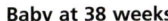

Baby at 38 weeks

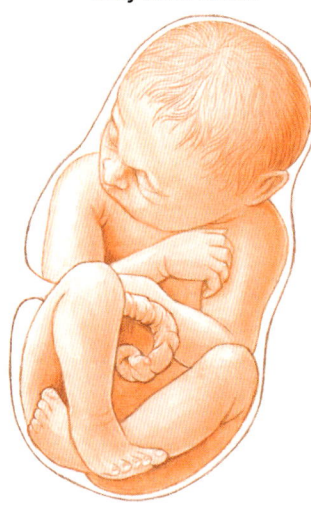

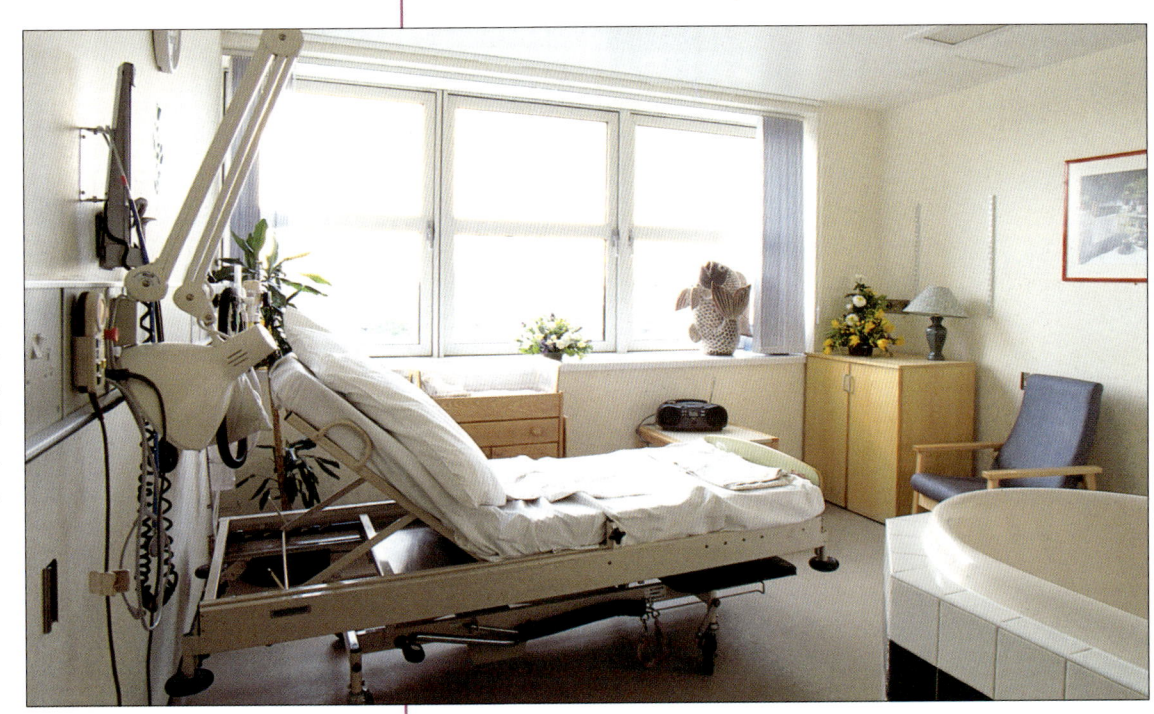

BIRTH DAY

THE DAY that your body has been gearing up for over the last nine months has almost arrived. You are ready to go at a moment's notice. If you can recognise the signs that indicate the onset of labour, and anticipate the sequence of events that make up the birth process, you'll feel much more relaxed, reassured and in control.

The early changes in your body that indicate labour is starting can take place over days without you being aware of them. The first sign is that your cervix softens ready for dilation (widening). True uterine contractions will start, but initially they'll be like the false Braxton Hicks' contractions you are used to, and you may not be able to distinguish them. As these early changes can be so subtle, your cervix may have dilated by as much as 2–3cm (around 1in) before you realise you are in labour. There are other key signs that the birth is about to occur.

A show

The neck of your uterus is sealed with a mucus plug that stops infection reaching the womb. As your uterus begins to contract, this plug will usually become dislodged, accompanied by some blood. This is called 'a show' and is a good indication that labour and birth are imminent.

However, a show can come days before labour actually starts, so it is advisable to wait until you are sure that true contractions have begun before going into hospital. You may feel a sudden urge to get to hospital as soon as possible, and this is perfectly understandable. But unless you have been advised to go straight away, it is usually better to wait out the opening stages of labour in the comfort of your own home.

Contractions

Labour has not officially started until you are having regular contractions, which dilate the

See page 89 for useful ideas on what to pack in your hospital bag for your time in hospital and your return home with your new baby.

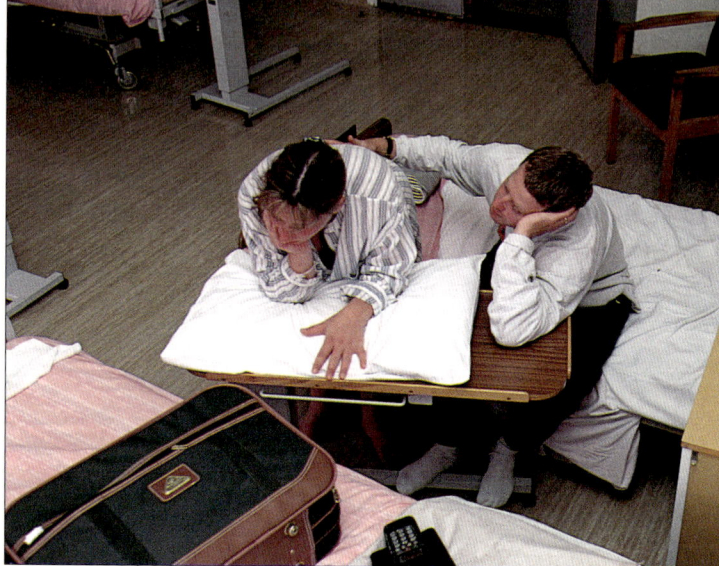

Labour lasts on average about eight hours, and is usually longer for first-time mothers. Be prepared for a long wait for both you and your partner.

cervix still further. The cervical opening must be at least 10cm (4in) wide before you can begin pushing. Labour contractions come in waves, getting faster and stronger as labour progresses.

You are usually advised to go into hospital once your contractions are coming every five minutes. For some women this can happen in just two hours, but for others it may take up to twelve hours to reach this stage.

Labour can be a long and tiring process, so although you may not be feeling very hungry at this time try to have some high-energy snacks and drinks to keep your blood sugar levels up and help avoid becoming dehydrated.

Waters break

As the baby's head presses against the opening in your cervix, the amniotic sac containing the amniotic fluid will rupture. This is what is meant by 'waters breaking' and can be a sudden burst, with gushing water, or a slow trickle.

If you are not already on your way, you are usually recommended to go into hospital once your waters break, even if your due date is several weeks ahead. You and your baby are now more vulnerable to infection at this stage. Your doctor and midwife may also be concerned that the umbilical cord could get trapped, which could cut off the blood supply from the placenta and starve the baby of oxygen.

THE LAST LAP
Emotional climax to pregnancy

The last few weeks and months of pregnancy can be a trying time, especially in hot weather. It is quite usual to experience emotional ups and downs during this time.

• You may be having trouble sleeping, especially if your baby is very active. There is no easy solution to this, just make yourself as comfortable as you can and try to get as much rest as possible during the day.

• The very fact of still being pregnant can be a source of irritation. You are tired of being big, and just want the whole thing to be over, with your baby safely in your arms. Try to stay patient. Your estimated date of delivery (see pages 14 and 15) is only an approximation, and it could be up to two weeks past this date before the hospital feels it is necessary to induce the birth.

• You may be anxious about your waters breaking unexpectedly, or not being able to reach the hospital in time. Rely on your partner to reassure you, even if it means sending him out to check that there is petrol in the car for the hundredth time!

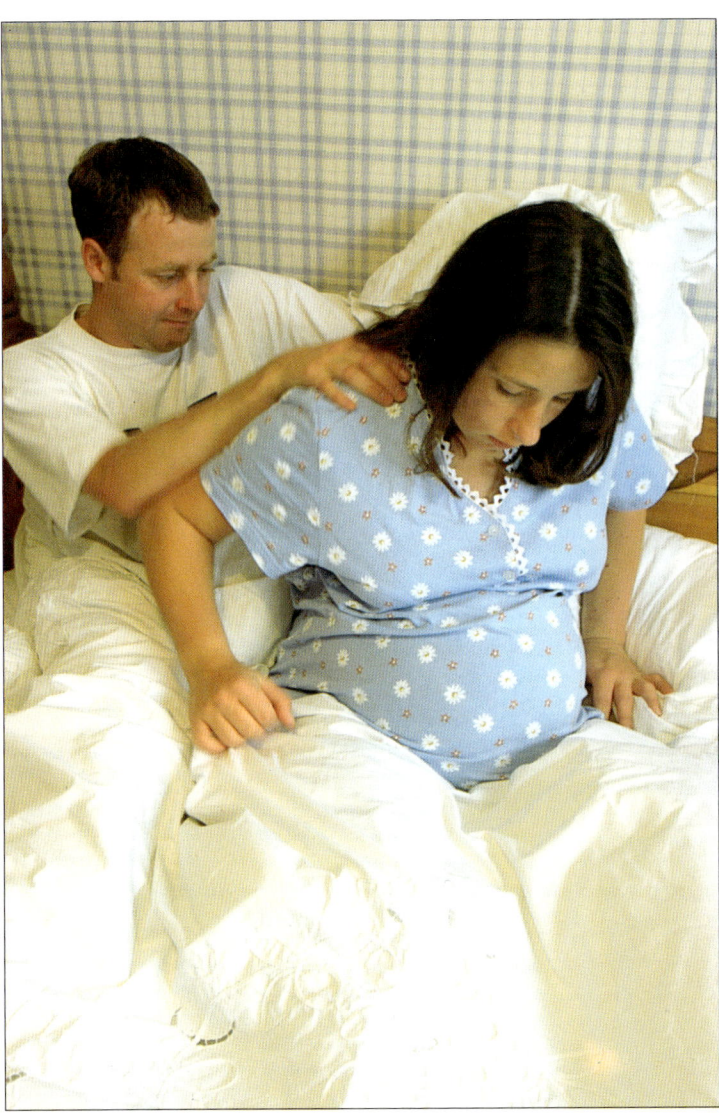

WEEK 39/40

After nine months of waiting, you'll soon be able to see your baby for the first time, and hold him or her in your arms! You should have your hospital bag packed and ready by the front door, and your partner on call to take you to the hospital and stay with you through labour.

What's happening to you
• Your breasts are starting to swell and fill with colostrum – your baby's first feed.
• Your cervix is softening in preparation to dilate so that your uterus can push the baby through your birth canal.
• You may be experiencing slight diarrhoea – this is just pre-birth nerves.
• You may feel a little unsure about your emotional state, and experience some mood swings. This is usually caused by the hormonal changes initiating the onset of labour.

for breastfeeding, which can start virtually the minute your baby is born.

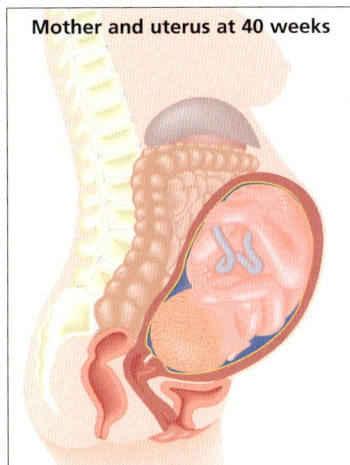

Mother and uterus at 40 weeks

What's happening to your baby
• Your baby is practising the 'rooting' reflex – moving the head from side to side while sucking. This is in preparation

• Your baby can gain as much as 225g (8oz) in weight per week in the last few weeks of pregnancy.

Placenta at nine months

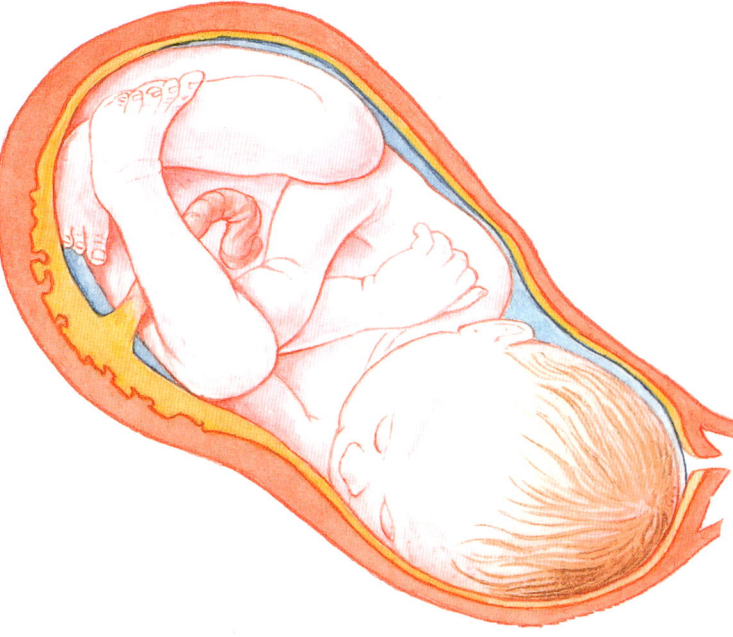

The placenta at 9 months is 20–25 cm (8–10in) wide and up to 2.5cm (1in) thick, a sizeable organ to support your baby in the womb.

*Y*OUR *B*IRTHPLAN

*G*ONE ARE the days when women in labour were only allowed to lie still and take orders. Now you are encouraged to consider all your options, decide what sort of delivery you want to have, and make sure everyone knows your preferences before labour starts. To help you to do this it is a good idea to write a birthplan.

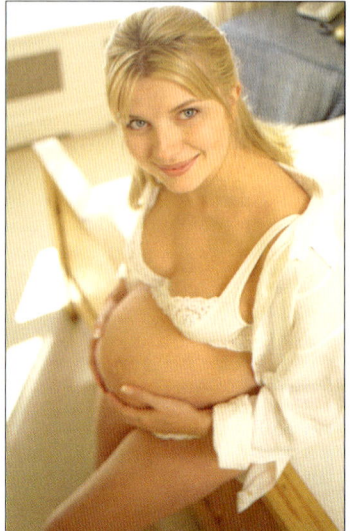

Labour is divided into three separate stages. The first stage is where the cervix softens, becomes thinner and opens wide (dilates) to enable the baby to pass through. The second stage is where the baby passes down the birth canal and is born. During the third stage, the placenta and amniotic sac are expelled from the uterus.

Labour is not over until after this third stage.

The birth process may not seem so clearly defined to you, however. The time taken to complete the first and second stages can vary enormously. For some women, these stages may be very drawn out, and yet for others it can all seem to happen in a rush. Many women do not even realise the third stage is happening as they are too preoccupied with holding their baby.

Your birthplan

Try to bear this in mind when devising your birthplan: you won't know for sure how long the various stages of labour will last, how tired you may get and how much pain relief you'll need. Try not to make your instructions too rigid and include a contingency plan so you have the flexibility to make last-minute changes. You should make sure your birthplan covers all the key issues, as follows…

Birth partner

Most women like to have someone they know with them during labour, apart from health carers. This is your birth partner, and could be your husband, partner or, if you prefer, your mother, sister or friend. If you want to have more than one person with you, you'll need to check with the hospital first as they'll have a limit on the number of people who can attend.

Examinations

If you would like your birth partner to be present during internal examinations, just say so. You'll probably have several examinations during the course of your labour.

Pain relief

Decide the level of pain relief you would like, and say which procedures you would prefer if extra relief is needed (see pages 90 and 91). Be prepared to be flexible, though. Everyone's pain threshold is different and you may well change your mind during labour.

Monitoring

Electronic monitoring is used for all high-risk deliveries and routinely for most normal deliveries (see pages 82 and 83). These machines provide an accurate picture of your contractions and the baby's well being, but they are not compulsory, so you don't have to give your consent.

Episiotomy

This is a simple incision intended to enlarge the vaginal opening to help mothers give birth more easily. A small cut is made in the perineum, the area of tissue between the vagina

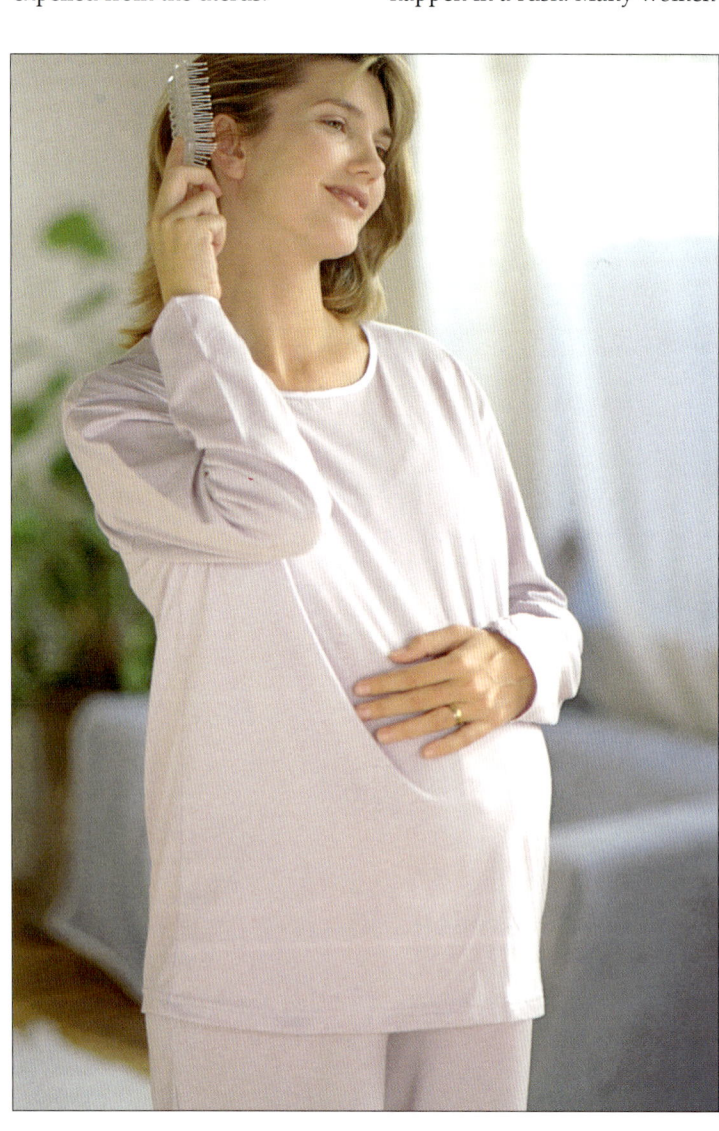

and anus. It is done under a local anaesthetic (the site of the incision is numbed with an injection) just before the baby is about to be born.

The advantage is that it prevents tearing and heals quickly. The drawback is that you'll need to be stitched immediately after the birth. These stitches can be uncomfortable for a few days. If you don't want an episiotomy, say so.

Birthpool

If you are considering a water birth (see pages 87, 89 and 91), you'll need to check with the hospital and start planning well in advance. Many hospitals have their own birthpool, but others do not, although they may allow you to bring one that you have hired. Some hospitals do not allow birthpools, however, usually because they lack available space.

Mobility

You'll find you are no longer confined to your bed during labour. Midwives believe that allowing mum to stay mobile until close to delivering makes for a quicker and happier birth. Pain relief – including a mobile epidural – is designed with this in mind. Some hospitals have radio-controlled monitors that do not require wires and so do not obstruct your mobility.

Birth positions

Moving around can make the contractions come closer together and gravity will help your baby descend through the birth canal more quickly. Many women say contractions are less

Your doctor or midwife will go over your birthplan with you to make sure they understand your requests.

Progress of labour – dilation of the cervix

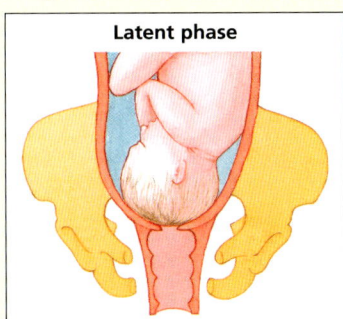 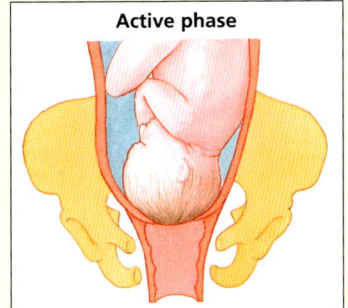 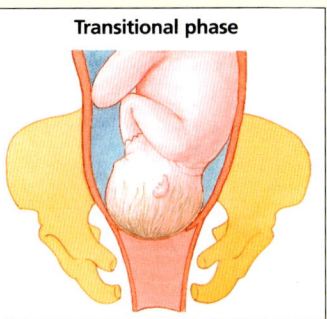

Latent phase — Active phase — Transitional phase

Each time you are examined, your doctor or midwife is checking to see how far your cervix has dilated. The opening must be 10cm (4in) before your baby can start to be born. The cervix thins and dilates a little more with each contraction. There are three distinct phases before full dilation is reached.
• Latent phase is when your contractions are just starting, and your cervix is starting to get thinner.
• Active phase is the widening when your contractions will become more intense and closer together.
• Transitional phase occurs just prior to delivery, and marks the end of the first stage of labour. Your cervix is now fully dilated, and your midwife will probably ask you to push with the next contraction.

painful when they are standing up so try to remain upright for as long as you can, leaning on your partner for support when you need it. You'll need to consider what position to adopt for the birth.

Standing

You could remain standing, supported by your birth partner to maintain your balance. Just holding on to him and moving around slowly rocking your pelvis will help. You can also lean forwards on to the bed and get your birth partner to rub your back to ease any aching.

Squatting

This position still allows you to use gravity. If your legs start to feel tired, get your birth partner to sit in a chair, then lean against him with his knees supporting your arms. You can also lean on a pile of cushions to help you keep your balance.

Kneeling

This position is easier on the legs than squatting, but you'll need some support to keep you as upright as possible as this position can be difficult to balance. The aim is still to let gravity help the birth, which will not happen if you go on to all fours during contractions. Try leaning on a chair, or get your birth partner to sit on the chair and lean on him so he can rub your back.

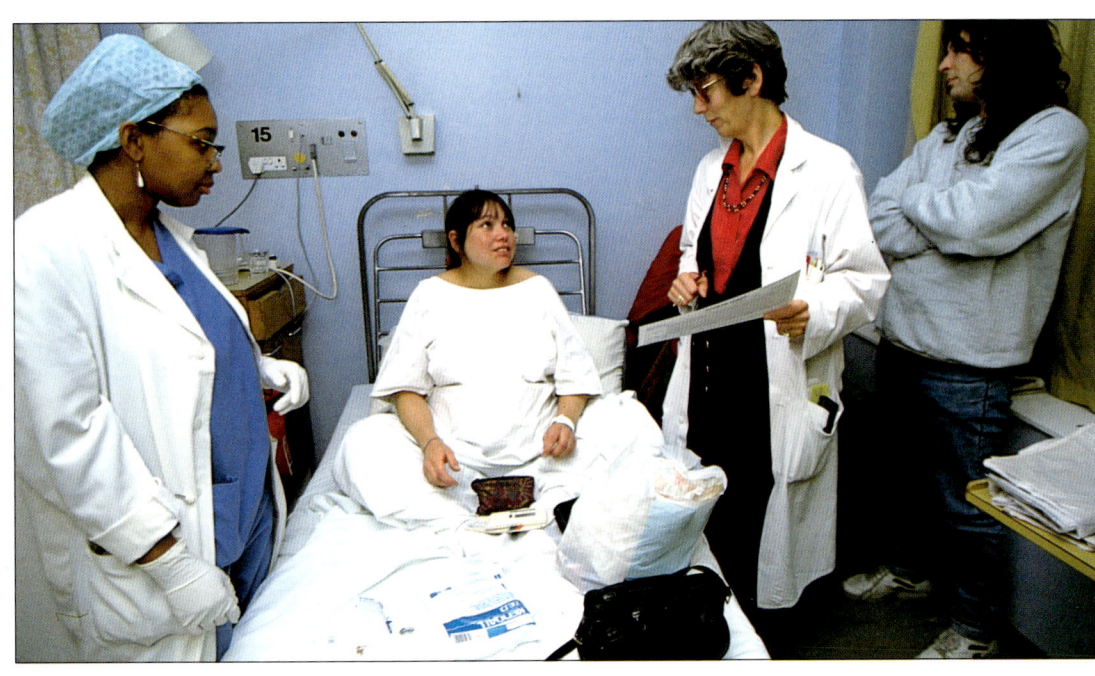

HOSPITAL ARRIVAL

AFTER MONTHS of preparation, your arrival at the hospital may seem an anticlimax. Where are the well-wishers, and the dozens of medical staff on hand to tend to your every need? The fact is that hospitals try to keep deliveries as low-key as possible so you can try to relax and concentrate on everything you've been told.

Although you are the centre of attention, you'll probably feel most comfortable if you are not surrounded by crowds of people, all trying to help or give advice. If your first stage (where your contractions come in waves) is very protracted, your midwife will probably leave you with your birth partner and simply check on your progress from time to time. The more space and quiet you have at this time the better.

Checking-in

Your midwife (or doctor) will need to assess your labour to find out how far you have progressed and what sort of delivery they can expect. Unless the labour is very long, you can expect the same midwife to be with you until delivery. You'll be taken to a private room where the midwife will read through your case notes, and ask you questions about the timing of your contractions and whether your waters have broken.

You'll then be given a gown. Most hospital gowns open at the back, which is not very convenient for breastfeeding. Ask whether they have front opening gowns if you intend to feed your baby straight after the birth.

Your midwife will feel your abdomen to ascertain the baby's position, and listen to the baby's heartbeat with a fetal stethoscope. She will also check your blood pressure, pulse and temperature, and a urine sample may be taken. An internal examination is then carried out to check how far your cervix has dilated. If it has reached 4cm (1 1/2 in) and your waters have not yet broken naturally, most hospitals will recommend that this is done artificially.

You will be offered a shower or a bath. Many women find that water is a great pain reliever. If your partner has remembered his swimming trunks, he can hop in with you to support you and rub your back.

Recognising contractions

Contractions feel like a strong tightening sensation under your 'bump' and in the small of your back, which lasts for a short while before being released. They are painful, and get more so as labour progresses. They help your cervix to dilate and enable the baby to descend the birth canal. It is only at this stage that you'll be asked to start pushing, and not before. Even if you feel the urge to push, it is important to wait for the midwife's directions as pushing too early will only tire you out and cause you to squeeze your baby unnecessarily.

You cannot control your contractions or get them to stop, and they will keep coming until the baby is born. At first, they will occur every 10–15 minutes or so and last up to a minute. As your labour progresses during this first stage (which can last for eight hours), your contractions will come faster – every 2–4 minutes.

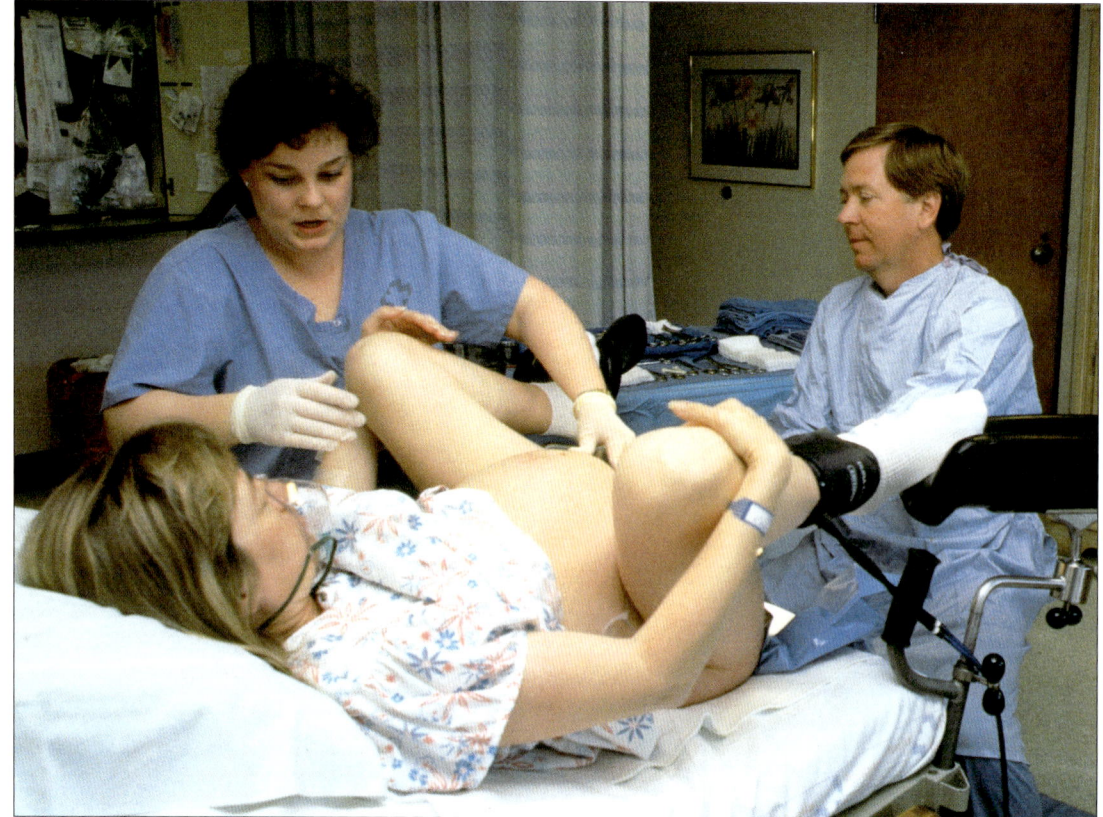

On average, first labour takes 14 hours from the first contraction. With a second child, it usually takes seven hours.

BIRTH PARTNERS
Providing help during labour

Today, most fathers choose to be present for the birth of their child. Despite the fact that many feel sick, faint and have difficulty seeing their partners in pain, most stay in the delivery room throughout labour. Many partners wish to play an active part in labour, helping mum with her contractions and breathing, and following the directions of the medical and midwifery staff. Others simply wish to sit by mum, mopping her brow and holding her hand to give comfort and support. Whatever their degree of involvement, it should not be forgotten that a partner's support is the assistance most often requested by women.

Water births are recommended heartily by those mums who try it. They say the water supports them and the pool makes them feel safe and protected.

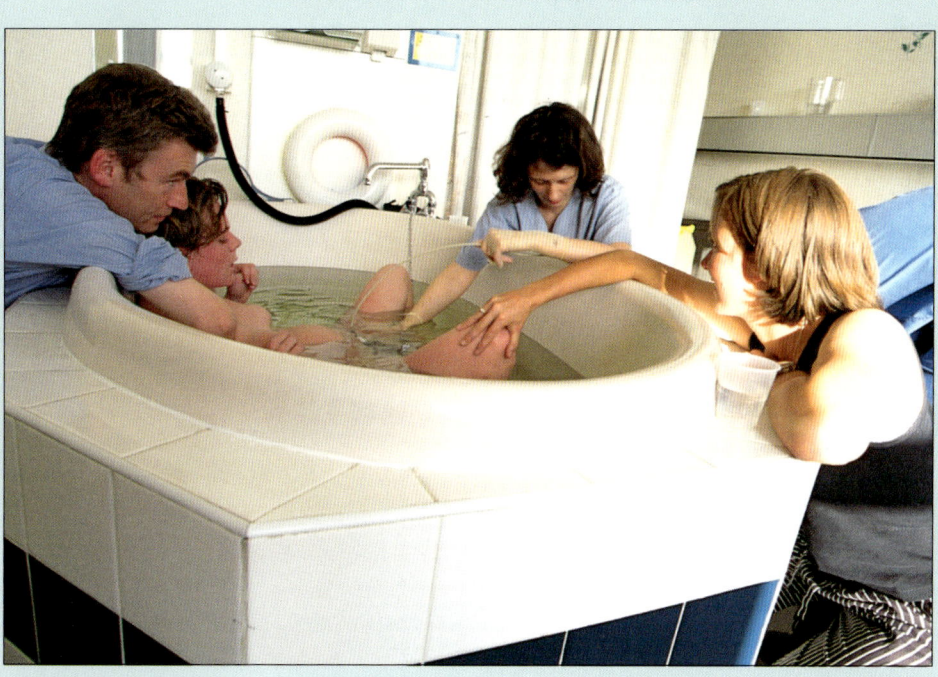

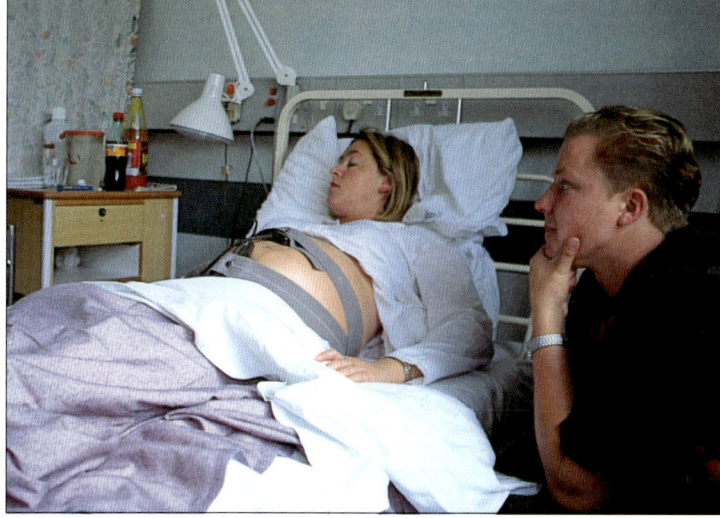

Having your partner with you during labour can be a great comfort, helping to alleviate some of the tension or anxiety you may be feeling.

At first, you may be able to manage your labour by getting your birth partner to support you, massage your back, and generally offer encouragement. Walk around if you like – motion and remaining upright help to speed up the process. It may help to listen to some music. Remember to eat and drink a little as you'll feel stronger and happier if you can keep your blood sugar levels up and avoid getting dehydrated.

The contractions will become most intense during the last few hours before delivery, and this is when you are most likely to want some form of pain relief (see pages 90 and 91).

Hospital Bag – deciding what to bring

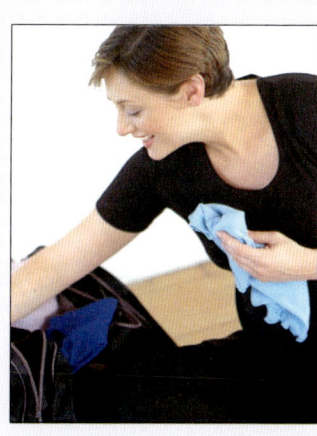

You may not use all – or any – of the items you take to hospital, but at least they are to hand if you need them.

- Comfortable top or nightshirt.
- Slippers.
- Music to relax you or provide a diversion.
- Sponges or a water spray to keep you cool.
- Lip salve in case your lips get dry.
- Massage oil.
- Snacks for energy.
- Camera to photograph the new baby.
- Hot water bottle to ease backache.
- Glucose drinks or fruit juice for energy and to keep you hydrated.
- Something for your partner to eat and drink.
- Earplugs for the postnatal ward (other newborns can be noisy).
- Sanitary pads.
- Telephone numbers and change for the public telephone (you won't be allowed to use a mobile telephone in the hospital).
- Baby clothes – a one-piece jumpsuit is usually sufficient.
- Nappies for the newborn.
- Carrycot and suitable car seat or harness for the journey home.
- Big and comfortable clothes to wear home.

PAIN RELIEF

EVEN IF you plan to give birth with as little medical intervention as possible, it is worth considering all your pain-relief options, and making sure there is something at hand. You may not feel you'll need drugs, but until you have been through labour you can't be certain how easy you'll find it to control the pain unaided.

As you approach the second stage of labour, when your baby is born, your contractions will get stronger and closer together. These contractions can be very intense, and so all women need some form of pain relief to help them cope. Even if you don't plan to use drugs, but prefer other alternatives, it is a good idea to look at all the methods of pain relief available to you in hospital.

Entonox

This is a mixture of nitrous oxide and oxygen, hence its other name 'gas and air'. It

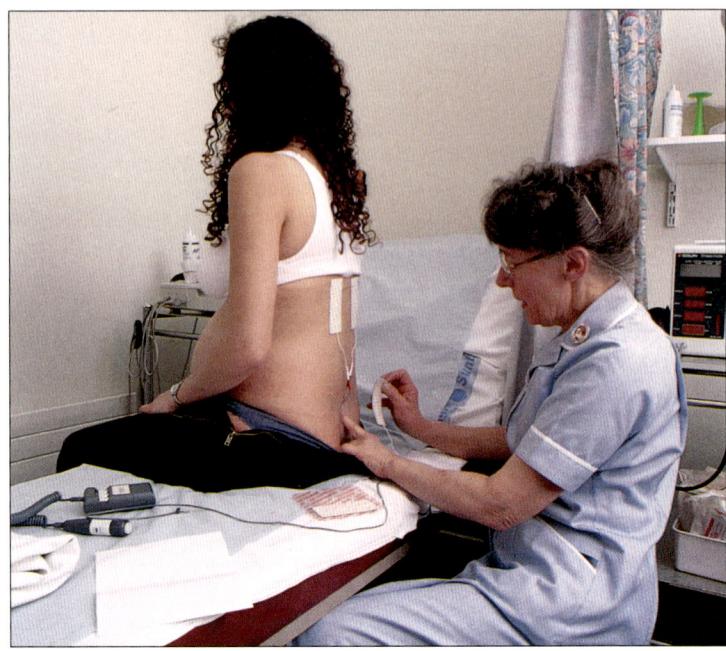

It is your responsibility to hire a TENS machine before the birth, so do this well in advance. They can really help during the first stage of labour.

works by numbing the part of the brain that registers pain, and produces a 'dizzy' sensation. It is available by the bed in the labour ward, and you'll be able to breathe as much as you want through a mask, even if you are having other forms of pain relief.

It works best if you take a few deep breaths of Entonox as soon as you feel contractions starting as it actually starts to take effect a few seconds later and lasts for about a minute at a time. The effect wears off quickly, however, and may not mask really strong pain.

Pethedine

This is a strong narcotic that is given via a single injection, usually into the thigh. It takes effect after a few minutes and lasts for a couple of hours. Pethidine can make you feel 'drunk' and you may lose perception of time. It is most

useful during long labours as it allows mum to get some sleep.

Pethidine can cross the placenta and affect the baby, however. If you are expected to deliver within four hours, some midwives may be reluctant to administer pethidine as it can affect the baby's breathing after the birth. Some women feel that the drowsiness it caused deprived them of the joyous experience of childbirth.

Epidural

Here, an anaesthetic is injected through a tube into the spinal column in the lower back. It works by blocking the pain signals from the cervix and lower body. The tube is usually left in place so that further doses can be given. It can only be carried out by an anaesthetist.

An epidural allows mothers a pain-free labour without making them feel drowsy or affecting the baby. It usually

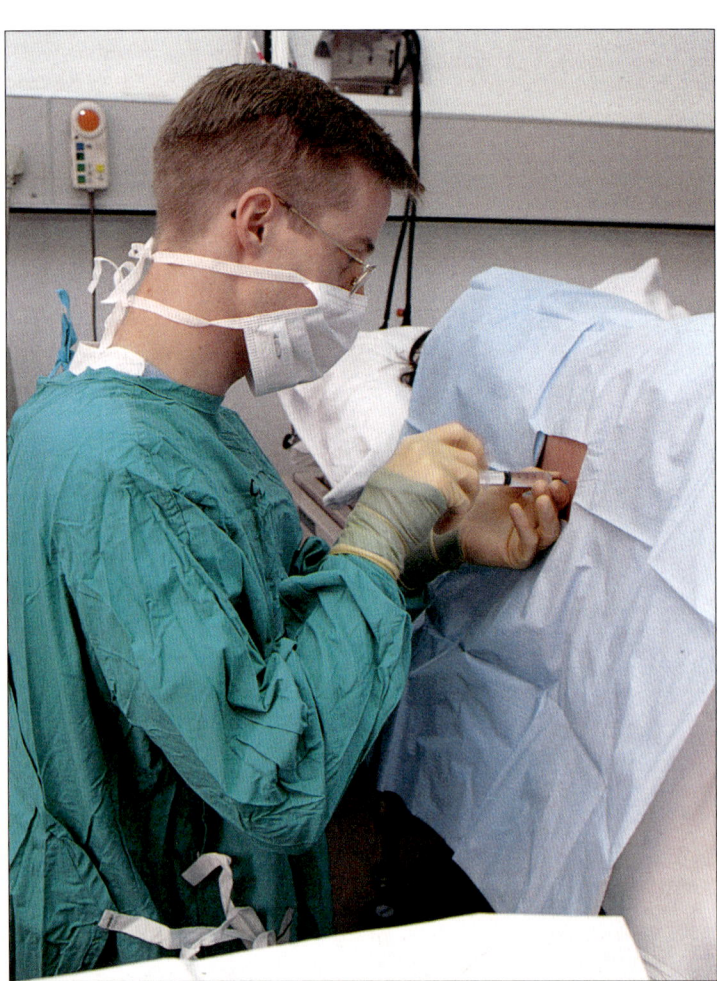

An epidural is the most effective means of pain relief, but it needs to be administered by an anaesthetist and may mean you cannot walk around.

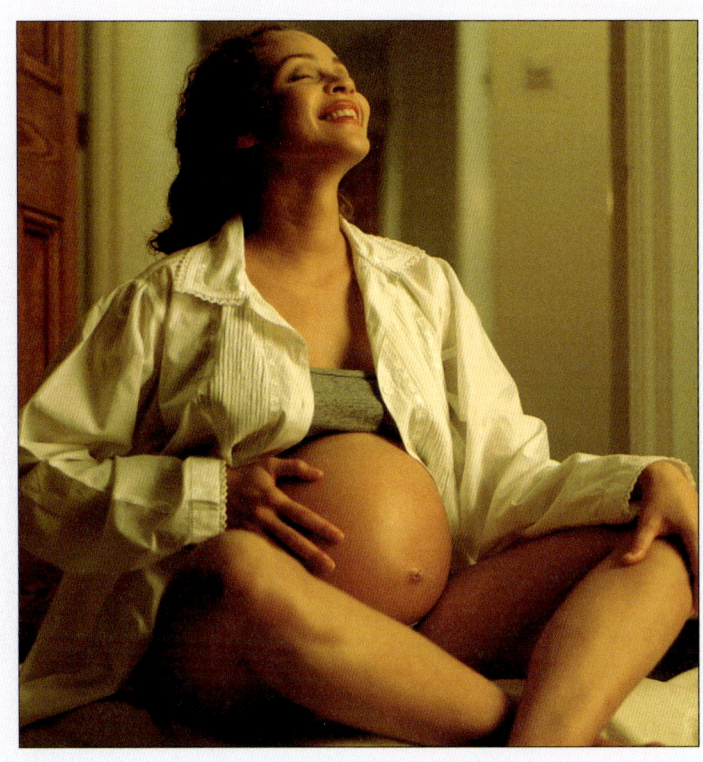

Alternatives – other forms of pain relief

There are other pain relief options that you might consider.

- **Active birth** is a system promoted by many people, including Janet Balaskas and Sheila Kitzinger, and classes are widely available. Women learn how to deliver their baby without drugs, using a combination of breathing and birth positions.
- **Water birth** has been promoted as a natural alternative, by Michel Odent, among others. Water not only helps relieve pain, it also provides buoyancy, which many mothers say makes them feel safer, and gives a feeling of privacy. Water is also thought to speed up labour and soften the perineum, so reducing the risk of tearing. Despite being called 'water birth', it is usually only employed for the first stage of labour.
- **Aromatherapy essential oils**, applied as a massage by a qualified practitioner, can relieve pain, relax the mother and hasten labour. Most hospitals will allow an aromatherapist to accompany you throughout labour.

Active birth techniques are more difficult to learn, and you will need to attend classes to practise the techniques, but many women say they found their active birth a very rewarding experience.

leaves them aware of contractions so that they can deliver normally. Epidurals are also effective for Caesarean sections, forceps deliveries and twin births.

In some cases, the anaesthetic effect may be too strong, and can stop you feeling the contractions. This can be a disadvantage during the second stage as you may not know when to push. Some mothers experience backache and headache afterwards.

Mobile Epidural

This is similar to a standard epidural, except that a different combination of drugs is used so that you can still walk around. This can provide a welcome relief, especially if you are experiencing a long labour. This method of pain relief is not available at all hospitals.

TENS

TENS (short for transcutaneous electrical nerve stimulation) involves tiny electrical impulses that are applied to the nerve fibres under the skin. It is designed for the first stage of labour only, but can be of great benefit, especially if this stage is protracted. It may have little effect during the second stage of labour, when the pain is usually too intense.

The TENS machine has four pads that are attached to your lower back, and linked to a battery-powered control panel. You can adjust the controls to boost the strength of the impulses and so increase the pain relief. Many women feel this gives them more control than other methods allow. If you want to use TENS you may need to hire a machine specially. Your midwife or doctor will tell you where to get one.

AFTER THE BIRTH
What can you expect

- The 'baby blues', is not uncommon in new mothers. Birth is an emotional time in itself, and you'll also experience major hormonal changes, as your body returns to its pre-pregnancy state. You may also be feeling exhausted, and anxious about your new baby. Trust your instincts, give yourself time to rest, and take advantage of any offers of help at this time. If your depression is very severe, or does not lift within a day or two, talk to your doctor.
- Bonding with the baby can happen more quickly with some mothers than others. Don't feel guilty if it doesn't happen immediately in your case – it soon will. Hold and rock your baby gently, and feed the infant. Once you get to know your baby your love will quickly grow.
- Breastfeeding can take place immediately after the birth, although some babies take a little while to learn how to latch on. There is a knack to getting the baby to take your nipple properly so that it can suck, but with a little patience this is a rewarding experience.

GLOSSARY

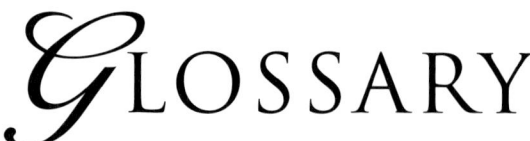

Amniocentesis
Test for fetal abnormalities. It involves the removal of a sample of amniotic fluid via a needle inserted into the mother's abdomen. It can detect chromosomal and genetic disorders.

Amniotic fluid
Fluid that surrounds and protects the fetus in the womb.

Anaemia
Reduction in blood levels of the oxygen-carrying pigment haemoglobin, usually due to iron deficiency.

Antibody
Chemical produced by white blood cells to fight infection. Also called immunoglobulin.

Antihistamines
Group of drugs used to treat severe vomiting in pregnancy and allergy symptoms.

Areolae
Dark area around the nipples.

Aromatherapy
Therapeutic use of plant oils. They are usually inhaled or applied to the skin, often by massage. When applied by a qualified therapist, they may help ease stress and pain in pregnancy and childbirth.

Bacteria
Microscopic organisms that can cause infection and disease.

Blastocyst
Cluster of rapidly dividing cells that forms early on in embryo development and implants in the lining of the uterus.

Braxton Hicks' contractions
Relatively painless contractions of the uterus that occur throughout pregnancy.

Breech position
A position in which a baby lies head upwards in the womb, rather than the usual head downwards, prior to birth.

Caesarean section
Surgical operation to deliver a baby via an incision in the abdomen. It is performed when normal delivery is not possible or would be more dangerous.

Calorie
Unit of heat energy, used to measure the amount of energy contained in food.

Cervix
Neck of the uterus (womb).

Chloasma
Mask-like area of pigmentation covering the nose, cheeks and forehead that can occur in pregnancy.

Chorionic villus sampling (CVS)
Test for fetal abnormalities. It involves the removal of small pieces of early placental tissue (chorionic villi) via a fine, flexible tube inserted through the vagina and cervix, or by a needle inserted into the abdomen. It can detect genetic and chromosomal disorders.

Chromosomes
Thread-like structures in the cells that contain the genetic code. Most cells in the body have 46 chromosomes.

Colostrum
Thick, yellowish, protein-rich fluid produced by the breasts for a few days after childbirth.

Cordocentesis
Test for chromosomal, genetic and other disorders, and infections in the fetus. It involves the removal of a sample of fetal blood via a needle inserted into the umbilical cord.

Dilation of cervix
Widening of the neck of the uterus to allow the baby to pass down the birth canal.

Diuretic
Drug that increases the body's output of urine. It is sometimes given to treat excess fluid in the tissues (oedema).

Down's syndrome
Chromosomal abnormality (47 chromosomes, instead of the normal 46) resulting in learning difficulties and some physical disorders. The risk of Down's syndrome increases with the age of the mother.

Ectopic pregnancy
Fertilised egg that implants outside the uterus, usually in a uterine (fallopian) tube. It requires emergency surgery.

Endometrium
Lining of the uterus.

Entonox
Painkiller, in gas form.

Embryo
Term for a baby during the first 10 weeks of development, after which time it is called a fetus.

Epidural
Short for epidural anaesthesia, a form of pain relief in which anaesthetic is injected into the space around the spinal cord.

Episiotomy
A cut made in the perineum (tissue between the vagina and the anus) to facilitate delivery and prevent tearing.

Fetal monitor
A machine often used during delivery to check the baby's heart rate.

Folic acid
Vitamin that plays a vital part in early fetal development. In its natural form, in food, it is known as folate.

Fraternal twins
Non-identical twins formed from separate eggs and sperm.

Rubella (German measles)
Virus that can cause serious fetal abnormalities if contracted during early pregnancy.

Hormones
Chemical messengers that are released into the blood and trigger a wide range of physical and emotional changes.

Identical twins
Twins formed when a single fertilised egg splits into two.

Implantation
Process by which a blastocyst attaches to the uterine wall.

Kangaroo care
Care of premature babies by close physical contact with the mother.

Kick chart
Record of fetal movement in the womb, usually taken over a 12-hour period.

Lanugo
Fine hair that covers the fetus.

Linea nigra
Dark line that often forms on a pregnant woman's abdomen.

Listeria
Bacterium found in dairy foods and meat that can lead to miscarriage and may be life-threatening in pregnancy.

Meconium
Dark substance passed in a baby's first bowel movement.

Miscarriage
Loss of the fetus before the 24th week of pregnancy. Also called spontaneous abortion. After this time, loss of the fetus is known as stillbirth.

Mucus plug
Blockage that forms at the cervical opening to protect the uterus from infection.

Oedema
Excess fluid in the tissues.

Oestrogen
Hormone responsible for female characteristics which (with progesterone) prepares the body for pregnancy.

Ovaries
Glands responsible for egg production and the release of oestrogen and progesterone.

Pelvic floor
Muscles and ligaments at the base of the abdomen that support the reproductive organs, bladder and rectum.

Pethidine

Powerful painkilling drug sometimes used in labour.

Placenta

Organ that allows oxygen and nutrients to pass from mother to baby, and allows waste products to be removed.

Pre-eclampsia

A serious condition in pregnant and post-natal women indicated by high blood pressure, oedema and protein in the urine. If untreated, it can lead to seizures (eclampsia).

Progesterone

Hormone that (with oestrogen) prepares the uterus for pregnancy.

Quickening

First movements made by the baby in the womb that the mother is aware of.

Resuscitaire

Resuscitation trolley holding equipment to help babies with breathing difficulties.

Rooting reflex

Instinctive way a newborn baby turns the head and opens the mouth when hungry and searching for the nipple.

Special care baby unit (SCBU)

Hospital unit devoted to the care of premature, underweight and sick babies.

Spina bifida

Defect in the development of a baby's spinal column, sometimes linked to folic acid deficiency.

Spotting

Appearance of small amounts of vaginal blood.

Term

Average length of time a baby spends in the womb.

TENS machine

A machine that helps ease pain by means of electrical impulses applied to the skin.

Triple test

Test for fetal abnormalities by analysing levels of three chemicals in the mother's blood.

Toxoplasmosis

Parasitic infection contracted from pet faeces, soil and undercooked meat that can harm a developing fetus.

Ultrasound Scan

A monitoring device that uses sound waves to produce an image of the baby in the womb.

Uterine tubes

Two tubes that carry eggs from the ovary to the uterus and where fertilisation occurs. Also called fallopian tubes.

Uterus (or womb)

Organ that houses the fetus during pregnancy.

Ventouse

Suction cup sometimes used to assist delivery.

Vernix

Waxy substance that coats the fetus in the womb.

Waters breaking

Rupture of the amniotic sac, which usually marks the onset of labour.

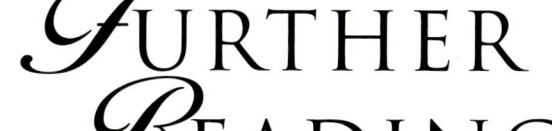

FURTHER READING

Bury, B. & Fowler, R. *Imaging Strategy, A Guide for Clinicians* (Oxford Medical Publications, 1992).

Close, S. *Birth Report* (National Foundation for Educational Research, 1980)

Clubb, Dr E. & Knight, J. *Fertility, A Comprehensive Guide to Natural Family Planning* (David & Charles, 1992).

Cooper, Dr C. *Twins and Multiple Births: the essential parenting guide from pregnancy to adulthood* (Vermilion, 1997)

Cutrona, Prof C. E. *Social Support in Couples* (Sage, 1996).

de Crespigny, L. & Dredge, R. *Which Tests for My Unborn Baby?* (Oxford University Press, 1996)

Donaldson, J. *Living with Asthma and Hay Fever* (Penguin, 1994).

Glade, Dr B. C. *Your Pregnancy Week by Week* (Element, 1999).

Glenville, Dr M. *Health Professionals Guide to Preconception Care** (Foresight: The Association for the Promotion of Preconceptual Care, 1998).

Kitzinger, S. *The New Pregnancy and Childbirth* (Penguin, 1997).

Mehta, D. K. (executive editor) et al *British National Formulary 37, March 1999* (BMA/Pharmaceutical Association of Great Britain, 1999).

Nolan, M. *Being Pregnant, Giving Birth* (HMSO/National Childbirth trust, 1996)

Pinkus, S. (editor) et al *The Modern Woman's Body* (Index, 1996).

Polunin, M. *Healing Foods* (Dorling Kindersley, 1999).

Stoppard, Dr M. *New Pregnancy and Birth Book* (Dorling Kindersley, 1999).

* *Advice and literature on preconception and pregnancy care are available from Foresight, telephone: 01483 427839.*

INDEX

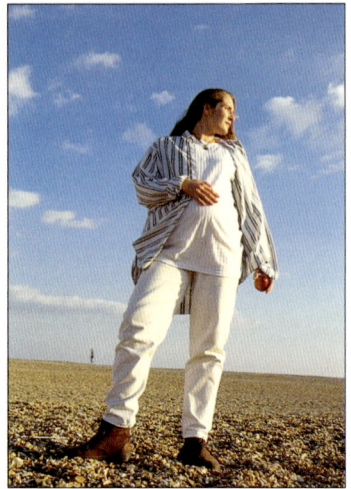

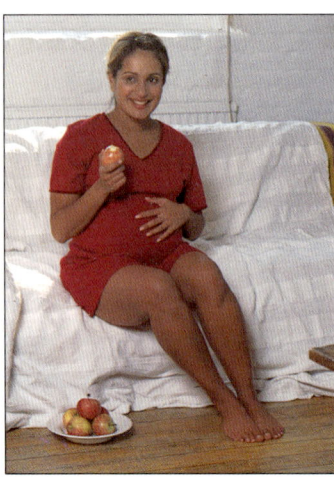

*Y*OUR *P*REGNANCY *D*IARY

Month 1

Month 2

Month 3

Month 4

Month 5

Month 6

Month 7

Month 8

Month 9

PREGNANCY MAGAZINE

Pregnancy and birth for mothers-to-be

'the clearest and most down-to-earth pregnancy magazine I could find'

'a real breath of fresh air – I wish I'd bought one earlier!'

This is the fastest-growing pregnancy magazine in the UK. Launched in 1997, it has quickly become a favourite with first-time mums-to-be due to it's practical and simple advice. It's aim is to unravel the sometimes mystifying medical issues and jargon that surround your pregnancy, as well as offering the whole host of extras you would expect from a leading glossy newsstand title:

• birth stories, telling you what the experience is really like
• feature covering up-to-the-minute issues that affect each and every pregnancy
• special practical birth section, covering your pain relief options, delivery procedures, essential advice to prepare for birth, and your birth choices
• news on the latest baby and pregnancy products
• the latest maternity fashion
• product reviews for the essential items you'll need to buy before delivery

Only £2.60, available bi-monthly at all good newsagents and supermarkets.

BABY'S BEST BUYS

The ultimate equipment guide for parenting

'I didn't realise how much was on offer – it's amazing what you can buy for babies now!'

'It's a real minefield out there – spending more doesn't mean you get better products, so it's important to do your homework'

Parents are now spending more than ever on baby equipment. This isn't just because they want the best for their baby – they're absolutely essential. So how does a first-time buyer know what makes a good highchair? Will your car seat work when he's two years old? What's the difference between a travel system and a three-in-one pram? You'll find these answers and much, much more in Baby's Best Buys:

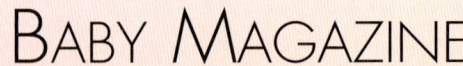

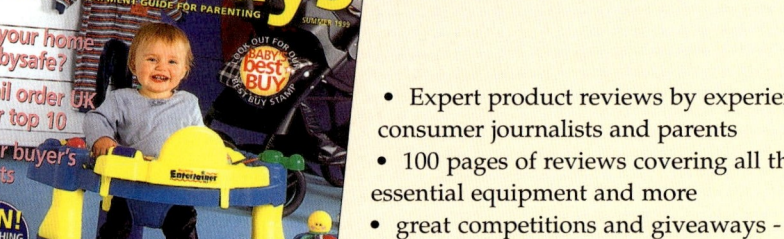

BABY MAGAZINE

Pregnancy, birth and babycare for first-time mums.

'the most interesting and helpful baby magazine I could find'

'a real wealth of information, and more like a friend than a magazine'

Baby Magazine, which has been going for over ten years, offers real insight into the world of parenting. With experts on hand to dispense practical parenting and medical advice for first-time mums, this magazine is a must for anyone new to the world of babies.

• in-depth features covering everything from nappies to breastfeeding to coping with sleepless nights
• the latest in baby news in the UK and abroad, from medical issues to new equipment
• reader's medical queries answered by our staff of doctors
• product reviews covering the latest baby equipment from bottles to prams to car seats
• fashion for baby and for pregnant mums
• essential contacts for parents to help you find the right service
• great competitions and giveaways – over £5,000 on offer every month
• fantastic subscription offers, like nappy disposers and baby monitors

Only £2.20, available monthly at all good newsagents and supermarkets.

• Expert product reviews by experienced consumer journalists and parents
• 100 pages of reviews covering all the essential equipment and more
• great competitions and giveaways - try your luck at winning everything you'll need to set up your nursery
• Prams, car seats, travel systems, strollers, cots, playmats, highchairs, dummies, bottles, teats, maternity bras, sterilisers, three-wheelers, nappies, pram shoes, baby clothes, changing tables, playpens, baby sun protection, non-biological washing powders...

Only £2.50, available at all good newsagents and supermarkets.

To find out more about *Baby Magazine*, *Pregnancy Magazine* or *Baby's Best Buys*, please call WV Publications on 0171 331 1000